POCKET GUIDE TO CHIROPRACTIC SKELETAL RADIOGRAPHY

Notice

Medicine is an ever-changing science. As new research and clinical experience broaden our knowledge, changes in treatment and drug therapy are required. The authors and the publisher of this work have checked with sources believed to be reliable in their efforts to provide information that is complete and generally in accord with the standards accepted at the time of publication. However, in view of the possibility of human error or changes in medical sciences, neither the authors nor the publisher nor any other party who has been involved in the preparation or publication of this work warrants that the information contained herein is in every respect accurate or complete, and they disclaim all responsibility for any errors or omissions or for the results obtained from use of the information contained in this work. Readers are encouraged to confirm the information contained herein with other sources. For example and in particular, readers are advised to check the product information sheet included in the package of each drug they plan to administer to be certain that the information contained in this work is accurate and that changes have not been made in the recommended dose or in the contraindications for administration. This recommendation is of particular importance in connection with new or infrequently used drugs.

POCKET GUIDE TO CHIROPRACTIC SKELETAL RADIOGRAPHY

Rhonda J. Boone, RT, DC
The Pain Center
Rosharon, Texas

With one chapter by
Lawrence H. Wyatt, DC, DACBR
Texas Chiropractic College

McGraw-Hill
Medical Publishing Division

New York   St. Louis   San Francisco   Auckland   Bogotá   Caracas
Lisbon   London   Madrid   Mexico City   Milan   Montreal   New Delhi
San Juan   Singapore   Sydney   Tokyo   Toronto

McGraw-Hill

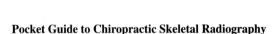

A Division of The *McGraw·Hill* Companies

Pocket Guide to Chiropractic Skeletal Radiography

1 2 3 4 5 6 7 8 9 0   DOCDOC   0 9 8 7 6 5 4 3 2 1 0

ISBN 0-8385-8130-7

This book was set in Times Roman by The Clarinda Company.
The editor was Steve Zollo.
The production supervisor was Catherine H. Saggese.
Project management was performed by Andover Publishing Services.
The cover was designed by Aimee Nordin.
R.R. Donnelley & Sons was the printer and binder.
This book is printed on acid-free paper.

Many illustrations in this book were taken from *Radiographic Anatomy &
Positioning: An Integrated Approach,* by Andrea Gauthier Cornuelle and Diane H.
Gronefeld, copyright © 1998 by Appleton & Lange.

Library of Congress Cataloging-in-Publication Data

Boone, Rhonda J.
    Pocket guide to chiropractic skeletal radiography / Rhonda J. Boone.
      p. : cm
    Includes bibliographical references and index.
    ISBN 0-8385-8130-7 (alk. paper)
    1. Radiography in chiropractic—Handbooks, manuals, etc. 2.
Skeleton—Radiography—Handbooks, manuals, etc. 3. Spine—
Radiography—Handbooks, manuals, etc. 4. Skeleton—Diseases—
Diagnosis—Handbooks, manuals, etc. 5. Title.
    [DNLM: 1. Musculoskeletal System—radiography—Handbooks. 2.
Arthrography—Handbooks. 3. Bone and Bones—radiography—Handbooks.
4. Chiropractic—Handbooks. 5. Extremities—radiography—Handbooks.
6. Radiography—methods—Handbooks. 7. Spine—radiography—
Handbooks. WE 39 B724p 2001]
RZ251 R33 B66 2001
616.7'107572—dc21

                                   00–032879

CONTENTS

PREFACE

Pocket Guide to Chiropractic Skeletal Radiography was written with the student chiropractor as well as the practitioner in mind. It is a "how to" reference guide that presents the reader with a wide range of essential information, from setting exposure factors and positioning the patient, to evaluating the x-ray film to ensure its diagnostic quality and estimating the cost of supplies and equipment.

The book is divided into two parts. The first four chapters provide basic information on the x-ray tube and ancillary equipment, on radiographic techniques and exposure factors, on developing the x-rays, on radiation safety, on quality control tests that can be done by the radiographer to ensure better diagnostic films, and on how to set up an x-ray suite and dark room. The next six chapters include descriptions of radiographic terminology and guidelines for the correct positioning of the patient. The information in these chapters is presented in concise outline form to make it easy for the student to learn the material and to allow practitioners to use the material as a quick reference guide. The following topics are discussed for each radiographic position: anatomy that should be included on the view; indication as to why the film is taken; recommendations on film size, tube tilt, and film focal distance (FFD); safety measures that should be taken, including collimation and gonadal shielding; patient position; location of central ray; recommended respiration instructions for the patient; and helpful hints.

These six chapters utilize a consistent format. The text is presented in outline form on the left-hand pages, and the right-hand pages contain clinical photographs demonstrating correct patient positioning, along with normal x-rays for abnormality comparisons. The patient is shown in an upright position whenever possible.

The final chapter, Chapter 11, defines advanced imaging modalities and explores how each can be used by the doctor of chiropractic. These modalities include computed tomography, magnetic resonance imaging, radionuclide bone imaging, and Doppler ultrasound. There is also an Appendix, which includes an equipment malfunction checklist and sample forms for the technical control of the radiologic suite.

Rhonda J. Boone

POCKET GUIDE TO CHIROPRACTIC SKELETAL RADIOGRAPHY

1

INTRODUCTION TO RADIOGRAPHIC IMAGING

X-ray machines contain three parts:
1. Generator
2. X-ray tube
3. Control console

GENERATOR

The generator supplies electrical power to the x-ray tube for production of x-rays. There are three types of generators:

- **Single-phase generator:** This generator requires the most amount of radiation to produce x-rays. It therefore exposes the patient to more radiation than does a high-frequency machine. This machine is obsolete due to new technology.
- **Three-phase generator:** This generator was developed to handle heavier loads of work (i.e., in a hospital or large outpatient setting). It requires less radiation to produce an image and exposes the patient to less radiation than does a single-phase generator. The motivation to produce or purchase this machine was the longer life of the x-ray tube (due to less heat production), making it more cost effective. The increased safety for the patient was a coincidental benefit.
- **High-frequency generator:** This generator requires the least amount of radiation to produce a diagnostic image, making this most recent development a better choice than the single- and three-phase generators.

X-RAY TUBE

Glass Envelope

- Made of hard heat-resistant glass to tolerate increased pressure and heat. The glass tube is not uniform in thickness. It is thinner at the exit window to avoid a decrease in intensity of the x-ray beam.
- Contains the vacuum necessary for x-ray production.
- Supplies a degree of electrical insulation.
- Assists in the removal of heat from the anode, preventing tube damage.

Tube Exit Window

- The useful beams of x-rays are emitted from the tube through the exit window.
- The glass envelope at the exit window is much thinner to minimize the reduction of the x-ray beam intensity.

Tube Housing

- The x-ray tube is securely positioned within a protective metal tube housing, giving mechanical support and protection for the x-ray tube.

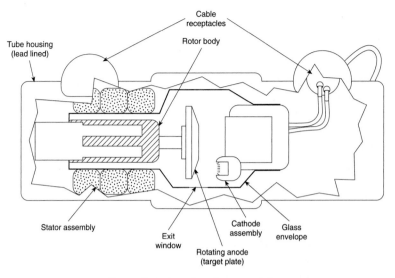

Figure 1–1. Drawing of an x-ray tube.

- The tube housing is made of steel or aluminum and is x-ray-proofed with lead.
- Within the housing, oil surrounds the tube to provide electrical insulation and remove heat generated by the tube.

Cathode
- The cathode is the negative electrode; it consists of small and large filaments inserted in a metallic focusing cup.
- The current that controls the heating of the small and large filaments in the tube is measured in milliamperes (mA). Thermionic emission is the term for the boiling off of electrons that occurs in the tube.
- Large filament is used with higher mA stations (150, 200, 250, 300, 500, 700, and 1000) where a larger number of electrons are required; less detail is recorded on the image at these stations.
- Small filament is used when a lower number of electrons are required, such as at 50 and 100 mA stations; at these stations, more detail is recorded on the film. The small and large filaments are placed in a focusing cup to control the divergence of the electrons.
- Small filament/small focusing cup produces a small focal spot on the anode, which creates an image with greater detail. Large filament/large focusing cup requires a larger focal spot on the anode, which decreases image sharpness on the film.

Anode

- The anode is the positive side of the x-ray tube, and the target plate for electrons to strike.
- There are two types of anodes, stationary and rotating. A rotating anode provides a larger surface area (125 times more) for heat dispersion.
- The quantity of heat produced at the anode is determined by kilovoltage (kVp), mA, and time. A high mA produces more heat at the cathode, boiling off more electrons; a longer exposure time allows more time for heat to be produced; and a high kVp produces a stronger positive charge, pulling the electrons across a gap to the target plate.

Target Plate Angulation

- The line-focus principle is used to provide a large area of heat distribution (to preserve the life of the x-ray tube) and a small focal spot to increase image sharpness. See Figure 1-2.
- The target plate (anode) is slanted at angles ranging from 7° to 20°.
- When the anode is tilted a small amount, the electron beam is distributed over a larger area of the target plate (actual focal spot), which aids in heat dispersion. From the plane of the film, it appears that the electrons strike a smaller area of the target plate (apparent focal spot), and this increases image sharpness.
- The most common anode angulation is 12°.

Anode Heel Effect

- The strength of the x-ray beam is not uniform as it travels towards the patient.
- The radiation intensity on the cathode side is stronger than on the anode side. This is because x-rays emitted on the anode side of the target must traverse a greater thickness of the target material than the x-rays emitted on the cathode side. See Figure 1-3A.
- The smaller the focal spot, the larger the magnitude of the anode heel effect.
- The longer the film focal distance (FFD), the smaller the magnitude of the anode heel effect. See Figure 1-3B.
- The anode heel effect can be used to benefit the operator by pointing the cathode (stronger intensity) towards the thicker body part. For example, while performing thoracic spine x-rays, the anode should be towards the cervical spine and the cathode towards the thoracolumbar spine. While performing femur x-rays, the anode should be towards the knee and the cathode towards the femur.

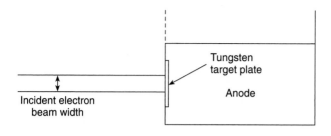

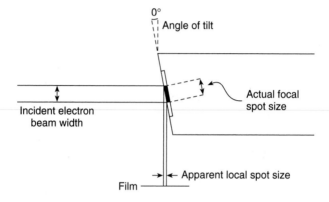

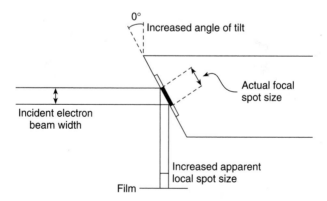

Figure 1–2. Anode with angulation demonstrating actual and apparent focal spots.

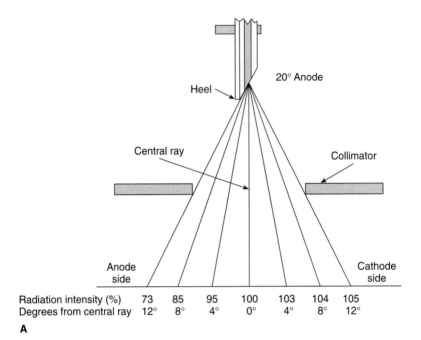

Radiation intensity (%)	73	85	95	100	103	104	105
Degrees from central ray	12°	8°	4°	0°	4°	8°	12°

A

B

Figure 1–3. A. Anode heel effect; the intensity of the x-ray beam increases toward the cathode. **B.** Increasing the film focal distance (FFD) results in less variation of the x-ray beam.

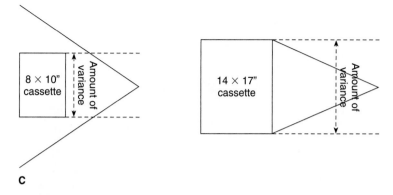

Figure 1–3. C. Anode heel effect; smaller film sizes result in less variation of the x-ray beam.

CONTROL CONSOLE

- This apparatus allows the operator to control the x-ray tube current and voltage so the useful x-ray beam is at proper intensity and penetrability to produce a diagnostic radiograph.
- **Line voltage compensator (surge protector):** A fluctuation in power voltage as low as 5% can affect the quality of the radiograph. The line voltage compensator prevents power surges while taking x-rays.
- **kVp:** Kilovoltage is selected by two adjustment knobs. Make major kVp changes in increments of 10 and minor kVp changes in increments of one or two, depending on the machine being used.
- **mA (millamperes):** The mA determines the exact amount of current used to heat the filament. Small filament consists of 25, 50, and 100 mA stations. Large filament consists of 150, 200, 300, and 600 mA stations. Small filament produces more detail on the film, but it increases the amount of radiation to the patient.
- **Timers:** Mechanical timers have minimal time of 1/4 second. Synchronized timers have a time equal to 1/20 second. Impulse is the most common and most accurate timer and has a minimal time of 1/120 second.
- **Exposure switch:** Two steps are required to produce an x-ray. The first switch is referred to as the dead-man switch; it activates the x-ray tube. The second switch energizes the anode and cathode to produce x-rays. The first switch is held down until the ready light appears, prompting the operator to push the second switch simultaneously.

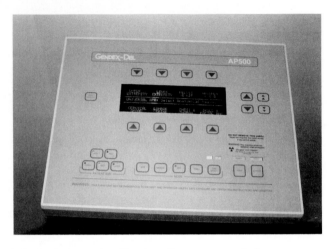

Figure 1–4. Control console with automatic exposure control. *(Courtesy of The Gilbert X-Ray Company of Texas.)*

ANCILLARY EQUIPMENT

Grids

- Lead strips arranged so that the useful radiation can reach the film and scatter radiation is absorbed by the lead strips.
- Used on body parts measuring more than 12 cm. in thickness (as the body gets thicker, more scatter radiation is produced).
- Improve film contrast by preventing scatter radiation from reaching the film.
- Three types of grids are available:
    1. *Parallel:* Lead strips are placed parallel to each other.
    2. *Focused:* Lead strips are angled to allow convergence of the x-ray beam. This type of grid must be used with an exact FFD.
    3. *Crossed:* Two parallel grids oriented at right angles to each other.
- **Grid ratio:** The height of the lead strips divided by the distance between the strips. Grids with higher ratios are more effective in removing scattered radiation.
- **Grid frequency:** Number of grid strips per inch. The higher the grid frequency, the higher the radiographic technique required and the greater the dose of radiation to the patient. (Remember that the grid is located behind the patient, so the patient receives the full dose of radiation and the film receives only the radiation that travels through the grid.)

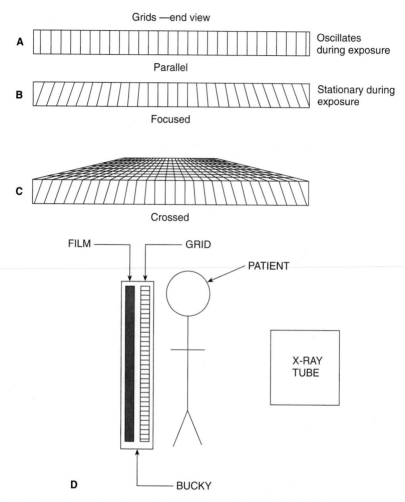

Figure 1–5. A. Parallel grid. **B.** Focused grid. **C.** Crossed grid. **D.** Placement of the grid between the patient and the film.

Collimator
- Device used to restrict the x-ray beam to the part of the body being examined.
- Increases film quality by reducing scattered radiation to the film.
- Decreases patient exposure to radiation by absorbing off-focus/scatter radiation. (Remember that the x-ray beam travels through the collimator before reaching the patient.)

- Allows operator to visualize how much of the body part will be included on the radiograph.
- Collimation is a source of radiation protection to the patient and many states have laws that require that collimation be visible on at least three sides of the film.

Film Identification

- The operator is responsible for providing a method of permanent identification to the film (name and date) before the film is processed (not handwritten on the film after it has been developed).
- A film flasher used in the darkroom is the most inexpensive but also the most inconvenient type of film identification. An automatic identification camera is the most convenient and may be used with the lights on in the examination room or the darkroom. (An automatic ID camera is recommended if there is more than one x-ray room sharing the same darkroom.)

Film Processors

- Three-minute tabletop processors are available. This processor will fit on the countertop and is adequate for most chiropractic practices. It requires less space and less volume of chemicals in storage containers, which decreases oxidation in a lower x-ray volume setting (such as that in a chiropractic office).
- Ninety-second processors are also available and are used in settings with a high volume of x-rays, such as a hospital. This processor is larger and requires more space to be installed.

Safe Light

- Light source placed in the darkroom.
- Must be placed 4 feet away from the working surface to avoid film fog.
- Contains a red filter over a fluorescent bulb to prevent light exposure to the film during developing.

Filtration

- Filtration is built into the machine and the amount is determined by the range of kVp required to produce radiographs.
- Selective filtration is added by the operator to enhance the appearance of a diagnostic film. This is most commonly used with thoracic spine films due to the variation in thickness at T1 versus T12. The filter is placed over the upper thoracic spine to prevent it from being too dark in radiographs taken at the exposure settings that will penetrate the lower thoracic spine.

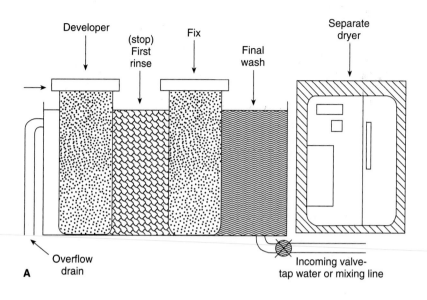

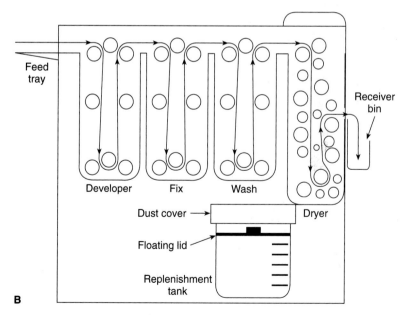

Figure 1–6. A. Manual processor. **B.** Automatic processor.

X-Ray Tables

- Tables are needed for taking radiographs that require the patient to be recumbent.
- Portable tables are available and recommended for chiropractic offices. They do not require as much space and can also function as an examination table.
- Stationary tables are also available. This type of table is bolted to the floor. Some have floating tabletops to move the patient without effort.

RADIOGRAPHIC
PRODUCTION

2

RADIOGRAPHIC FILMS, SCREENS, AND CASSETTES

Film Construction

- The film base provides a durable support for the photosensitive emulsion, which contains the actual image.
- The film base is a thin layer of polyester plastic that is light, flexible, and durable.
- A thicker base decreases image sharpness.
- Emulsion consists of a gelatin containing photosensitive compounds such as silver bromide and silver sulfide (referred to as silver halide crystals), which is placed on both sides of the base of the film.
- Silver halide crystals are sensitive to blue light.
- Rare earth screens emit green light so the film has a green dye added to it.
- It is very important that the film-screen combinations have matching color spectrums.

Types of Film

Screen Film

- Contains emulsion on both sides of the base of the film.
- Designed to be used with intensifying screens.
- Intensifying screens are made of fluorescent materials that produce light when they interact with x-ray photons.
- Single-screen systems (extremity cassettes) produce one image on one side of the film, which allows for greater detail.
- Regular cassettes contain two screens that produce two images, one on each side of the film, allowing the operator to decrease the patient's radiation exposure. However, some detail is lost because two images are superimposed on each other.

Duplicating Film

- Contains emulsion on one side of the film only.
- Used to make a copy of an original x-ray.
- It is placed on top of the film being copied. The correct order of the materials is light source, original film, and duplicating film, with the emulsion side of the duplicating film against the original radiograph.

Film Speed

- Faster film speed requires a shorter exposure time, which decreases the amount of radiation exposure to the patient; however, some detail is sacrificed.
- Slower film speed requires a longer exposure time, which increases the amount of radiation received by the patient; however, the detail is increased on the film.

- Detailed/extremity cassettes use the same speed of film as regular cassettes, but there is only one intensifying screen in the detailed cassette. This provides more detail on the film because of only one image produced (regular cassettes have two images superimposed). Since only one image is produced on the film, increased radiation is required, which increases radiation exposure to the patient. (Do not confuse this with film speed.)

Handling and Storage of Film

- Radiographic film is sensitive to temperature, humidity, pressure, light, and x-rays.
- High temperature may cause fog to be seen on the film after processing.
- High humidity may cause films to stick together or jam in the processor.
- Excessive light in the darkroom will cause fogging on the film, causing a washed-out appearance that results in decreased detail on the film.
- Storage should be temperature-controlled.

Cassettes

- Lightproof containers are used to protect and transport the x-ray film before and after exposure.
- Cassettes should be stored in an upright position to avoid pressure artifacts on the film inside the cassettes.
- Do not leave cassettes open. This allows artifacts to gather on screens as well as allows the screens to be damaged.

Intensifying Screens

- All cassettes have two intensifying screens, except for extremity cassettes, which have only one intensifying screen.

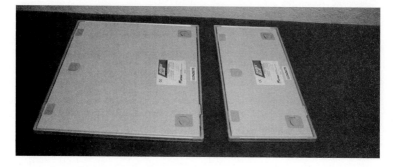

Figure 2–1. X-ray cassettes. *Left,* 14 × 17 inches; *right,* 7 × 17 inches.

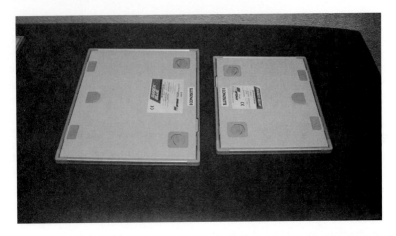

Figure 2–2. X-ray cassettes. *Left,* 10 × 12 inches; *right,* 8 × 10 inches.

- Extremity cassettes produce greater detail because only one image is produced on one side of the film. (All other cassettes produce two images superimposed on each other.)
- Intensifying screens should be labeled with a permanent marker to locate cassettes containing artifacts. (Place a number in one corner of the screen; if the number is placed in the center, it may interfere with anatomy on the radiograph.)
- Routinely clean screens with a lint-free cloth and a commercially produced screen cleaner.
- Life of an intensifying screen is approximately 7 years.

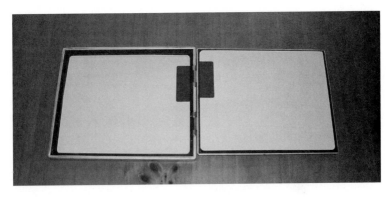

Figure 2–3. Intensifying screens inside a cassette.

MANUAL FILM PROCESSING
Following are the six steps in manual film processing.

1. Prewetting
- The film is placed in water in order to penetrate the emulsion so that it will take up the processing chemicals more rapidly and uniformly.

2. Developer
- In this stage, the silver ions of the exposed crystals are converted into elemental silver.
- The converted silver is concentrated in the region around the sensitivity specs.

3. Stop Bath
- Used with manual processing only.
- Consists of a tank of water in which the film is rinsed off to stop the action of the developer.

4. Fixing Agents
- This step is the clearing agent because it removes the undeveloped silver halide from the film.
- The fixing agents shrink and harden the emulsion.

5. Stop Bath
- In this stage, water is used to wash away fixing chemicals on the film.
- Poor washing of the film leads to poor archivability of the film (meaning that the film may turn brown or appear washed out over time).

6. Drying
- This is the last step of processing, accomplished by blowing clean, warm, dry air over the film. (Keep the drying area as clean as possible to avoid drying dirt and lint into the film.)

AUTOMATIC FILM PROCESSING
- Film is manually introduced into the processor.
- Rollers feed the film through the developer and fixer tanks and through the dryer.
- Movement of the film through the rollers removes the chemicals from the film (eliminating the stop baths needed in manual processing).
- Developer temperature depends on film type, the speed at which film moves through the developer, and formulation of the developer. (Obtain recommendation from the company that supplies chemicals and film.)

- Automatic processors require a constant flow of fresh water to properly wash the film. If the film comes out wet, make sure that the water to the processor is turned on.

RADIOGRAPHIC TECHNIQUES

Terminology

- **Density:** Overall blackness of the film.
- **Contrast:** Difference in optical densities (shades of gray). Allows for differentiation between anatomic structures. (Low contrast = many shades of gray; high contrast = black and white; high contrast is recommended for bone films and low contrast for soft tissue films.)
- **Detail:** Ability to visualize small anatomic structures.
- **FFD** *(film focal distance):* Distance from the x-ray tube target area to the film.
- **OFD** *(object film distance):* Distance from the object being x-rayed to the film.
- **Penumbra:** Blurred margin of an x-ray image.
- **Umbra:** Sharp margin of the image on the x-ray.

Kilovoltage (kVp)

- Indicates the penetrating power of the x-ray.
- Creates an electrical potential between the anode and cathode so the electrons from the cathode will travel to the anode.
- kVp is inversely proportional to contrast (high kVp = low contrast).
- To visualize a minimal change on the film, the kVp has to be changed at least 5% (approximately 4 kVp).
- To visualize a 50% change on the film, the kVp must be changed 15% (approximately 10 kVp).

Milliamperage (mA) and Seconds

- Controls the amount of heat produced at the cathode, which determines how many electrons are boiled off (thermionic emission).
- mA controls the density of the film.
- mA is inversely proportional to time (high mA = short exposure time).
- Seconds controls how long the cathode boils off electrons, so the combination of mA and seconds controls quantity of x-rays.
- Short exposure time decreases detail on film, provides decreased motion on the film, and decreases amount of radiation exposure to the patient.
- Example: 50 mA at 3/5 second and 300 mA at 1/10 second each produce 30 mAs (mA × s) at 70 kVp. A setting of 50 mA at 3/5 second produces more detail, more radiation exposure to the patient, and lower contrast than 300 mA at 1/10 second, which is a fast exposure time.

Focal Spot Size

- Small focal spot (target area on anode) corresponds with the small filament of the cathode, which corresponds with 50 and 100 mA stations.
- Small focal spots (50 and 100 mA stations) should be used with body parts measuring less than 12 cm. and should use less than 70 kVp.
- Large focal spot corresponds with the large filament of the cathode, which corresponds with 150 mA station or higher.
- Large focal spot (150 mA or higher) should be used with body parts measuring more than 12 cm. and should use 70 kVp or higher.
- In summary, large focal spot = high mA station = short exposure = less radiation to the patient = less detail on film.

Film Focal Distance (FFD)

- The most common FFDs are 40 in. and 72 in.
- A short FFD (40 in.) gives the patient less radiation but increases the amount of penumbra, which decreases detail.
- Short FFD increases magnification of the body part.
- Exposure factors must be increased by a factor of 4 when increasing from 40 in. to 72 in.

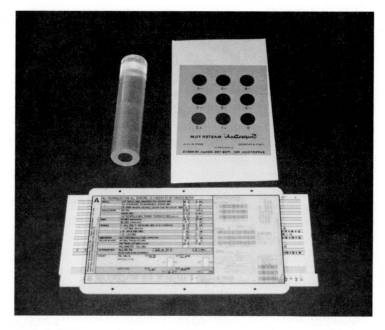

Figure 2–4. Manual calculator for setting radiographic technique. *(Courtesy of Supertech, Inc.)*

Supertech

- Slide rule that can calculate exposure factors.
- Recommended for people with little experience in setting exposure factors.
- Reduces the number of repeat films, which decreases radiation exposure to the patient.
- Requires the radiographer to identify a total correction factor for the x-ray machine being used. This is done only once, using equipment and instructions provided in the kit. After this is done, the radiographer measures the patient and places the measurements in the slide rule, selects a kVp and mA, and an exposure time is provided.

RADIOGRAPH EVALUATION

- The final stage of taking an x-ray is evaluating the image and deciding whether it is diagnostic (acceptable) or not.
- Proper ways to place films on the view box:
    1. *AP/PA films* should be placed on the view box as if the radiographer is looking at the front of the patient—a right marker on the film should be placed on the radiographer's left side.
    2. *Lateral projections* should place the film on the view box as if the radiographer is looking at the patient in the actual position.
    3. *Extremity films* of the fingers, hand, wrist, forearm, toes, and foot are placed with the digits pointing upwards. All other extremity films are placed with the digits pointing downward.
- The radiographer should scan the film and determine if it is too dark, too light, or diagnostic. On skeletal radiographs, the radiographer should be able to identify the cortex of the bone. On soft tissue films, the radiographer should be able to identify the different soft tissue densities (the soft tissues should not blend together).
- Overexposed films will be very dark, making it difficult to differentiate the anatomy. The radiographer must then make a decision on whether or not enough information can be obtained by using a hot light (a bright light held next to the film) or if another radiograph should be taken.
- Underexposed films will be very light with a washed-out appearance, making it very difficult for the radiographer to identify the cortex of the bone and/or the soft tissue densities.
- Proper patient identification (with ID camera—not handwritten with a marker) must be on the film, including the patient's name and date of the exam. A permanent right or left marker should be on the film (again, not handwritten).

- *All* anatomy of interest must be present on the film. If not, the film must *always* be retaken.
- The patient's position must be correct so the anatomy of interest may be visualized as close to reality as possible. This requires correct patient position, tube tilt, central ray, FFD, and OFD.
- Three sides of collimation must be visible on the film (often by state law). The radiographer should always use the maximum amount of collimation possible. It decreases radiation to the patient and increases film detail because it filters out scatter radiation. Collimation is the only device that provides only benefits. For example, increasing mA also decreases exposure time, resulting in decreased radiation to patient, but it sacrifices (decreases) detail on the film.

EFFECTS OF PATIENT STATUS ON RADIOGRAPHIC IMAGES

Four Body Types

1. Sthenic
- This is considered the average body build.
- The patient is generally physically fit and has good muscle tone and bone mass.
- This body type is the basis for established exposure factors.

2. Hyposthenic
- This is a more slender body build than sthenic.
- The patient is healthy but thin and somewhat underweight for height.
- Hyposthenic patients require fewer exposure factors than those with a sthenic body type.

3. Hypersthenic
- The patient has massive or heavy body build.
- This body type requires more exposure factors than the sthenic body type.

4. Asthenic
- The patient is slender and frail (common in elderly patients).
- The patient may be physically unfit and emaciated, usually as a result of pathology.
- This body type requires the least amount of exposure factors.

Disease Processes of the Skeletal System
- Osteolytic disease processes require a decrease in exposure factors.
- Osteoblastic disease processes require an increase in exposure factors.

- Skeletal radiography requires high contrast films (low kVp).
- When bone pathology is present, a change in kVp is required because of the need for a change in penetrating power.

Disease Processes of the Respiratory System

- Lung x-ray requires low contrast (high kVp, 100 to 120) to visualize bronchial markings (soft tissue).
- Lung pathology requires a change in mAs.

3

QUALITY CONTROL
AND RADIATION SAFETY

QUALITY CONTROL

Quality control appears to be the weakest link in the x-ray department. Every office that contains an x-ray room should develop a strong quality control program to ensure that the imaging system is functioning optimally. The following tests may be performed in the office.

Light Leak Test
- This test should be performed in the darkroom with all lights off and all doors closed.
- Allow eyes to adapt to the darkroom before searching for light leaks.
- Most common sources of light leaks include light fixtures, vent pipes, water pipes, sewer pipes, suspended ceiling tiles, improperly mounted pass boxes, and poorly fitting doors.
- Repair leaks that are identified and repeat the light leak test.
- A written record of location of light leaks and corrective action taken should be kept.
- This test should be done on an annual basis.

Film Fog
The two main sources of film fog in the darkroom are from light leaks and chemicals.

Testing for Film Fog without Special Equipment
- Close the darkroom and turn on the safelight.
- Lay a single sheet of film on the work surface.
- Immediately place a piece of cardboard over the film, leaving 2 in. exposed, and wait 5 minutes.
- Move the cardboard so that another 2 in. of the film are exposed and wait 5 more minutes.
- Move the cardboard so that another 2 in. of the film are exposed and wait another 5 minutes.
- Process film.
- Visually compare each 2-in. segment to the other for discrepancies. Only gross fog problems will be detected using this test method.

Testing for Film Fog with a Sensitometer
- This test requires a sensitometer and a densitometer.
- A *sensitometer* is a photographic device that places an image gradient of 21 different steps of exposure on the film.
- A *densitometer* is a device that reads the densities after the film is developed.
- Expose the sensitometer tablet on the film.
- Cover half of the tablet with a piece of cardboard while leaving the other half uncovered.

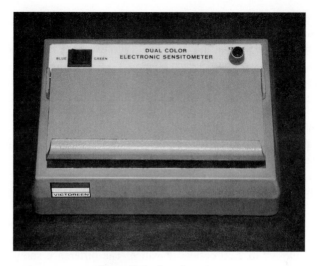

Figure 3–1. Sensitometer.

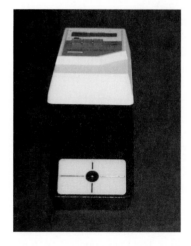

Figure 3–2. Densitometer.

- Wait 5 minutes and then process the film.
- Compare the optical densities of the two halves of each step of the sensitometer tablet with a densitometer.
- If no film fog is present, then the two halves should be within 0.02 optical density units of each other.

Chemical Fog Testing
- Remove two films from the film storage area.
- Process one film normally.

- Place the second film into the fixer, bypassing the developer.
- Measure the density of each film with the densitometer.
- If no film fog is present, the densities of the two films should be within 0.02 optical density units of each other.
- An elevation of density on a film that was processed only through the developer indicates there is fog on the film due to the developer.

How to Analyze a Sensitometer Tablet

- **Base plus fog:** Measured at step 1 of the sensitometer. Base plus fog value should not be above 0.30 optical densities.
- **Speed index/mid-density:** A step on the sensitometer tablet that yields a density of about 1.0 to 1.20 optical densities. This is usually step 10, 11 or 12. Use the same step each time the test is performed.
- **Contrast index/density difference:** The difference between the step that has a density of less than 0.45 optical densities and the step that has a density closest to 2.20 optical densities. The difference should be approximately 1.75 optical densities. Make sure that the same step is used each time the test is performed.
- **Processing temperature:** It is important that the same thermometer be used on a daily basis and placed in the same location in the tank.
- These tests should be performed on a daily basis and charted. If there is any fluctuation on the chart, it is an indication of a problem with the quality control program.

Processing Artifacts

Guide Shoe Lines

- Guide shoes are plastic devices that direct the film into the tanks of solutions.
- Guide shoes leave long marks that run the length of the film and are 1 in. apart.

Pi Lines

- Pi lines run at 90° angles to guide shoe lines. The lines appear 3.1416 in. apart. The lines run across the width of the film.

Crescent Moons

- Crescent moon marks are formed when the film is kinked or bent while unloading the cassettes and running the film through the processor.
- The film is much more sensitive after exposure.

Lightning Marks/Static Electricity

- Static electricity may appear due to humidity or carpet in the darkroom.
- The marks occur randomly on film.

Cassettes and Intensifying Screens

1. Identify each cassette.
   - Numbers should be written on the screens with a permanent black marker, preferably placing it on the top of the film and in one corner.
   - This is done to locate artifacts on specific cassettes.
2. Make sure the film used matches the color spectrum (green or blue) of the screen.
3. Make sure that good film/screen contact is uniform over the useful area of the screen.
   - This is tested by using a copper mesh wire placed between two pieces of plastic. The mesh wire is then placed over each cassette and exposed.
   - Poor film/screen contact will demonstrate areas of less detail of the mesh wire.
4. Screens should be cleaned quarterly with a cleaning fluid obtained from the manufacturer.
5. Do not leave cassettes open. This can attract foreign objects to the screen or damage the screens if anything is placed on top of the screen.
6. Screens should be replaced every 5 to 7 years.

X-Ray Output Linearity

- This test checks the calibration from one mA station to the next.
- This test may be done with an aluminum step wedge.
- A constant kVp and mA per second is used with a change in mA and time, to produce the same mA per second from one mA station to the next. (Example: at 70 kVp and 20 mA per second, 200 mA are produced in 1/10 second and 100 mA in 1/5 second.)
- X-rays of the aluminum wedge are taken at each mA station with the same kVp and mA per second and then compared from one film to the next. The density should be the same on each film.
- The test is more sensitive when a densitometer is used to measure the densities.
- Lack of linearity makes it impossible to develop a reliable technique chart.

Exposure Reproducibility

- This test checks several exposures (using the same mA, time, and kVp), to ensure that the same density is produced with each exposure.
- Testing is performed using an aluminum step wedge.
- Four exposures are made of the aluminum step wedge using the same kVp, mA, and time with each exposure (only the cassette is changed). The densities are then compared from one film to the next and should be the same.
- This test is more sensitive when a densitometer is used to measure the densities.

Timer Accuracy

- This test can be performed by a radiographer by using a spinning top.
- Place a cassette with a film in it under the x-ray tube.
- Place spinning top on film and make an exposure at a specific time (example: 1/4 second).
- Identify type of rectification for x-ray unit (ask dealer). Half-wave rectification will have 60 pulses/second, and full-wave rectification will have 120 pulses/second.
- Use the following formula to calculate actual time used: pulses/second × time = pulses.
- Compare number of pulses to number of dashes on the film. These should equal each other.
- If number of pulses on the film are less than pulses calculated by formula, then the timer is cutting off too early and the film will be underexposed.

Collimator Alignment

- Most state regulations require that collimation may vary no more than 2% of the source image distance for length and/or width.
- This test may be performed by placing a quarter in each corner of the collimation and exposing the film.

View Box

- All light tubes inside the view box should emit light of the same color.
- Light tubes should be the same intensity.
- Flickering fluorescent tubes must be replaced.
- The room in which interpretations are performed should be dimly lit so light does not interfere with the viewing of the films.

Regulation Requirements

Some states require that timer accuracy, exposure reproducibility, linearity, tube stability, collimation, and kVp accuracy be tested every 18 months. The measurement of kVp accuracy is an invasive procedure and should be performed by an x-ray physicist.

RADIATION PROTECTION

Maximum Permissible Occupation Dose

- This is a formula used to calculate annual and lifetime maximum doses. The formula is calculated as follows: (N-18)5REM, where *N* is the person's age in years and *REM* is the abbreviation for radiation equivalent to man.
- A person must be over 18 years old to perform x-rays.

• The formula states that you are allowed 5 REMs for each year of age above 18 years.

Personnel Monitoring

• All personnel exposed to radiation must wear a film badge to detect the amount of radiation exposure.
• Film badges are worn around the collar to avoid being covered by lead aprons.

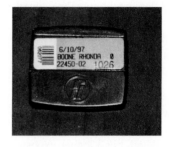

Figure 3–3. Film badge used for personnel monitoring.

• Regulatory authorities require some form of documentation for all personnel in the facility.
• A report of a high dose of radiation must be submitted in writing to the regulatory agency. A reason for abnormally high exposure must be included. The agency will consider changes if personnel were not actually overexposed, but changes are not often granted.

Time as a Protection Factor

• Time is a very inexpensive way to help control radiation exposure to the patient.
• The least amount of time used for exposure gives the patient the least amount of radiation exposure.
• Time is inversely proportional to mA. The higher the mA station, the less time of radiation exposure to the patient.

Distance as a Protection Factor

• The inverse square law states that the further one moves away from the source of radiation, the less intense the radiation level will be.
• This plays a major role in radiation protection, especially for the operator performing the x-rays.
• The operator should be at least 6 feet from the source of radiation. However, a lead apron should also be worn, or the operator should stand behind a protective wall when possible.

kVp

- Controls the penetrating power of the x-ray photons.
- It is important to use enough kVp to penetrate the body part being x-rayed.
- Optimal contrast is required on the film for correct diagnosis.
- A higher kVp allows for a lower exposure time to be used, which reduces patient radiation exposure.
- If kVp is too high, the film will be too dark and undiagnostic.

mA

- Determines the amount of electrical current flowing through the filament. Time and mA complement each other.
- The higher the mA station, the shorter the exposure time, giving the patient less radiation exposure. However, a higher mA station also causes less detail on the film.

Focal Spot

- This refers to the area on the anode from which the x-rays are emitted, as seen from the viewpoint of the film.
- The smaller the focal spot, the greater the detail, but a longer exposure time is required. This produces more radiation exposure to the patient. (A small focal spot corresponds with 50 and 100 mA stations, and a large focal spot corresponds with 150, 200, and 300 mA stations.)

Gonadal Shielding

- Heart-shaped gonadal shielding is used for females. The top of the heart should be placed at the level of the anterior superior iliac spine (ASIS).

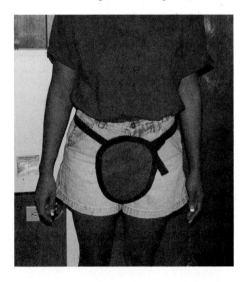

Figure 3–4. Gonadal shielding.

- Triangle-shaped gonadal shielding is used for males.
- Lead aprons should be used if someone is holding the patient.
- Gonadal shielding should not be superimposed over anatomy of interest on the film.

Grids and Bucky Devices

- The use of grids requires more radiation exposure to the patient (the grid is between the patient and film); however, it filters out scatter radiation from the film, producing a better quality film that is more diagnostically useful.

Holding Patients

- The operator and/or physician should never hold a patient if at all possible.
- Mechanical devices should be used as a first choice.
- If mechanical devices are not available, a person (1) not at risk for occupational exposure, (2) not pregnant, and (3) over 18 years of age should be utilized.

Radiography during Pregnancy

- If at all possible, do not x-ray a pregnant patient.
- Radiation exposure during the first trimester is more dangerous to the fetus than exposure during the second and third trimester, with the third trimester being the least dangerous.
- Female patients within the childbearing age range should be asked if there is a possibility of pregnancy. If there is a chance of pregnancy, two methods may be used. A pregnancy test may be ordered or the 10-day rule may be used. The rule states that a female of childbearing age should only be x-rayed during the first 10 days following the onset of menses. (Ordering the pregnancy test is often more practical, especially if the patient is injured.)

Protective Devices

The following is a list of devices that decrease the amount of radiation exposure to both the patient and the operator.

1. *Film/screen systems:* The higher the film speed combinations, the lower amount of time required. This decreases radiation exposure to the patient and operator.
2. *High-frequency generators:* This type of generator requires less exposure time to produce a diagnostic x-ray, decreasing the amount of radiation exposure to the patient and the operator.
3. *Collimation:* Decreases secondary radiation to the patient and operator as well as scatter radiation to the film.

4. *Gonadal shielding:* Whenever possible, gonadal shielding should be used to protect the reproductive organs; however, gonadal shielding cannot be used if it will be superimposed over the part of interest being x-rayed.

5. *Gloves and apron:* Whenever possible, gloves and/or an apron should be worn to decrease radiation received by the operator and/or patient.

Operating and Safety Procedures

Regulating authorities require that each x-ray facility have a written operating safety procedures manual that includes the following:

1. Applicable regulations for the facility.
2. List of individuals who are authorized to order x-rays.
3. List of individuals who are authorized to take x-rays.
4. Description of personnel monitoring systems, provisions for wearing the monitors, and reports of doses.
5. Directions on how to operate x-ray machines in the facility.
6. Specification for processing the film.
7. Description of quality control programs and tests established for the facility.

4

INITIAL SETUP OF THE RADIOLOGIC SUITE

DESIGN AND PLACEMENT OF THE X-RAY SUITE
- The x-ray suite should be placed in an area of the office with the least amount of traffic of people. This will decrease the amount of lead shielding required in the walls.
- The x-ray suite needs to be located near incoming electrical power and water supply.
- The x-ray tube, when possible, should be placed where exposure is directed towards an outside wall. This will decrease the amount of lead shielding required in the walls.
- Use a space large enough to obtain a 72-in. film focal distance (FFD), which is required for lateral views of the cervical spine and chest x-rays. Space may also be needed for an x-ray table if extremity exams will be performed.
- The larger x-ray room requires less lead shielding in the walls because of the distance between the primary beam and the wall. It is recommended that a radiation physicist calculate the amount of lead shielding required.

DESIGN OF THE DARKROOM
- The darkroom needs to be large enough for the processor, chemicals, film bin, utility sink, and darkroom technician.
- Good ventilation is needed due to the strong chemicals.
- A floor drain is required for the processor.
- A water source is required for the processor and for the utility sink used for cleaning the processor.
- Adequate electrical outlets are needed for various pieces of equipment (i.e., processor, film identification flasher, and safelights).
- The darkroom must be light-free.
- *Do not* carpet the darkroom. Carpet contributes to static electricity artifacts on films.

EQUIPMENT RECOMMENDATIONS
- When deciding on new or used equipment, consider the long-term costs and radiation exposure to patients.
- When buying new equipment and supplies, it is recommended to choose one company. Each company develops equipment, film, and chemicals that will be most efficient working in conjunction with each other.

Generators
- The choices are single-phase, three-phase, and high-frequency. Single-phase generators require the most lead shielding in the walls because they produce more scatter radiation.

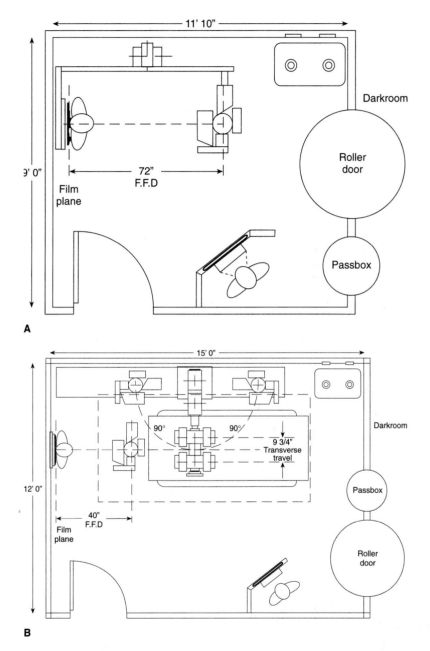

Figure 4–1. A. Example of x-ray room design with upright Bucky only. **B.** Example of x-ray room design with table and upright Bucky.

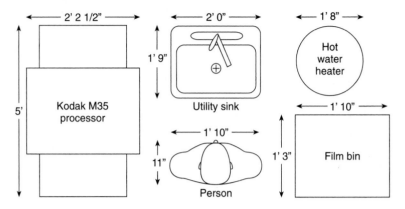

Figure 4–2. Example of darkroom design.

- High-frequency generators produce less scatter radiation, requiring less lead shielding in the walls.
- Three-phase generators fall between the other two.

Film/Screen Combinations
- The choices with rare-earth cassettes are 100 to 1200 speed.
- The faster the film speed, the less radiation required, which decreases the amount of lead shielding required (but less detail is obtained).
- Another consideration when choosing film speed is the type of x-rays performed. Recommended film/speed combinations for skeletal radiography are 400 to 600 speed, but may vary with the different manufacturing companies.

Recommended Maximum mA and kVp Capabilities
- Maximum mA and kVp capabilities recommended for skeletal radiography are 300 mA and 125 kVp. The greater the capacity of the equipment, the more shielding required.

STATE REQUIREMENTS
Requirements vary from state to state, and you should contact your state association and regulatory authorities for specific requirements. Most states require each office to have a policy and procedures manual and a radiation protection program. The states' primary concern is that the patients and operators are receiving the least amount of radiation possible while producing a diagnostic image.

The policy and procedures manual should include the following:
1. How personnel monitoring will be done and record keeping procedures.

2. Directions on how to operate the equipment in the facility.
3. Specifications on who may order x-rays and who may take the x-rays.
4. Specifications on processing time and temperature for the processor.
5. Description of the quality control program with what tests are performed, how often tests are performed, and description of record keeping of the tests.

Figure 4–3 contains a radiation program recommended by Gilbert X-Ray Company of Texas. Each office will need to adapt a radiation safety program and safety procedures manual to accommodate their facility.

RADIATION PROTECTION PROGRAM

The Operating and Safety Procedures are available for any or all employees. It is strongly suggested that employees review and become familiar with these procedures on a yearly basis.

A. **Personnel Monitoring**

  1. _____ badges are used in this facility and the badges are changed every _____.

  2. A control badge is provided by _____ and kept _____.

  3. Always wear your personnel monitoring badge when you are working and make sure it is the badge assigned to you. Wear the badge on your collar. When you wear a lead apron, the badge should be on the outside of the apron. Employees should leave their badge at work before leaving each day to avoid possible deceptive exposure reading.

  4. There will be no minors allowed to work in the radiation area.

  5. Use gloves, aprons, etc. Try to keep your personnel radiation exposure to a minimum. Be aware of where you are standing, and how long you stay in the radiation area. Do not enter or remain in a radiation area unless it is necessary, and remember, time, distance, and shielding are your best factors to help safeguard yourself from excessive radiation exposure. If an employee is working in more than one facility it is up to them to notify the R.S.O. The R.S.O. will be responsible to notify that facility to get a copy of the dosimetry reports to ensure that the employee does not exceed 5 rem of occupation exposure per year.

Figure 4–3. Example of a radiation protection program. *(Courtesy of The Gilbert X-Ray Company of Texas.)*

6. When you must hold a patient, use gloves and aprons, or get a family member to hold for you.

7. If you suspect there has been an excessive exposure or a radiation incident, immediately notify _____, the R.S.O.

8. Should an employee become pregnant, please notify _____, the R.S.O., immediately in writing with the date of conception. At that time an additional badge will be ordered for that employee to wear at abdominal level to monitor fetal dose.

B. Quality Assurance Programs

1. Quality Control is done _____ on the processor. _____ is responsible for doing quality control testing. A monthly computerized graph with the quality values plotted is kept in the quality control notebook. The corrective actions are noted on the graph itself or under the deviations tab of the notebook.

2. An _____ month Preventative Maintenance and Calibration will be done on the x-ray machine. All documentation on the calibration will be in the blue notebook provided by Davenport X-Ray Co., Inc. A PM and calibration sticker with the date of the current PM and calibration and the next PM and calibration due date will be placed on the x-ray machine.

3. The protective devices will be checked annually and results kept in the State Compliance notebook by the R.S.O.

C. Training

1. The R.S.O. will be responsible for the training of all the personnel not holding a license from the A.R.R.T.

2. All personnel with a license from the A.R.R.T. will provide copies of all Continuing Education certificates to the R.S.O.

3. A review of the "Operating and Safety Procedures" and the "Radiation Protection Program" will be completed upon employment, by the R.S.O.

D. Posting and Labeling

1. All entrances to the Radiation Area will be posted with a "Caution Radiation Area" sign.

2. All x-ray machines will be labeled with a sticker, stating that when the machine is energized it produces radiation.

Figure 4–3. *(continued).*

3. The R.S.O. will check that all the necessary signs and labels are in place when he or she does the yearly audit.

E. **Compliance with Dose Limits to the Public**

(The highlighted method is the one that pertains to this facility).

1. The room survey has been performed by a physicist; that information is kept by the R.S.O.; that information can be found _____ .

2. The room survey is being done by using a quarterly film badge system.

3. A drawing of the x-ray room and the nonradiation areas, with each nonradiation area badge and its number, will be kept by the R.S.O.

4. Upon completion of the room survey, the yearly calculated dose for the nonradiation areas will be kept by the R.S.O.

F. **Inspections/Audits**

1. A quarterly review of the Operating and Safety Procedures and the Radiation Protection Program will be done with all employees. These will be checked and updated during the yearly audit conducted by the R.S.O.

EMPLOYEE SIGNATURE   DATE   R.S.O. SIGNATURE

Figure 4–3. *(continued).*

Table 4–1 lists some typical costs of supplies so that an estimated cost of overhead may be calculated.

TABLE 4–1. X-RAY COST EXAMPLES

X-Ray Film	Size	Cost/box of 100	Cost/sheet
	14″ × 17″	$129.00	$1.29
	10″ × 12″	$ 68.00	$ .68
	8″ × 10″	$ 45.00	$ .45
Chemicals	Developer	$23.95 per 5 gal.	
	Fixer	$16.95 per 5 gal.	
Casettes with Screens	14 × 17	$262.50	
	10 × 12	$157.50	
	8 × 10	$120.00	
	14 × 36	$675.00	
Other Supplies	Thickness caliper	$25.95	
	Lead apron	$170.00	
	Gonad shield	$ 87.00 (set of 2)	
	Manual ID printer	$159.00	
	R and L markers	$ 9.95 set	
	Stainless steel therm.	$ 37.95	
	Safe light	$ 82.95	
	Bright light	$ 69.95	
	Viewbox 14 × 17 (single)	$119.00	
	Viewbox 14 × 17 (3-bank)	$195.00	
	Film storage bin	$195.00	
	Sensitometer	$675.00	
	Densitometer	$795.00	
	Film duplicator	$535.00	
	Silver recovery system	$ 79.00	
	X-ray filter kit	$795.00	
	Film filing folders 14 × 17	$ 9.35/50	
	10 × 12	$ 6.25/50	
	8 × 10	$ 5.75/50	
	Supertech (complete kit)	$109.00	
	ID cards	$ 60.00/1000	
	Extremity support table	$195.00	

Courtesy of the Gilbert X-Ray Company of Texas.

5

INTRODUCTION TO RADIOGRAPHIC POSITIONING

RADIOGRAPHIC TERMINOLOGY

- **Projection:** The path of the x-ray beam as it exits the x-ray tube and passes through the patient.
- **Position:** The placement of the patient's body.
- **Anatomic position:** The patient is in an upright position, arms slightly abducted, palms forward and feet directed straight ahead.

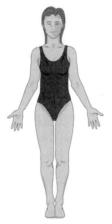

Anatomical position

- **Supine:** The patient is lying on the back, face up.

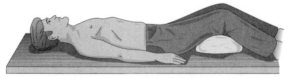

Supine (dorsal recumbent) position.

- **Prone:** The patient is lying on the abdomen, face down.

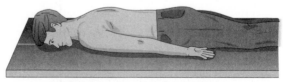

Prone (ventral recumbent) position.

- **Erect:** The patient is in the upright position.
- **Recumbent:** The patient is lying down in any position.
- **Oblique:** Between an AP or PA projection and a true lateral projection.
- **Left posterior oblique position (LPO):** The left posterior aspect of the body is closest to the Bucky.

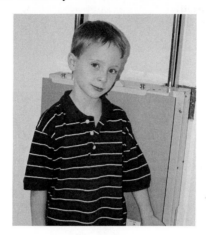

- **Right posterior oblique position (RPO):** The right posterior aspect of the body is closest to the Bucky.

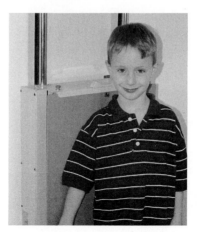

- **Left anterior oblique position (LAO):** The left anterior aspect of the body is closest to the Bucky.

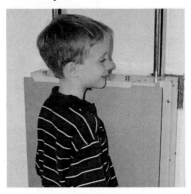

- **Right anterior oblique position (RAO):** The right anterior aspect of the body is closest to the Bucky.

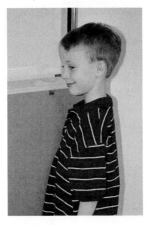

- **Anterior or ventral:** Referring to the front half of the body.

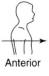
Anterior

- **Posterior or dorsal:** Referring to the back half of the body.

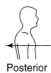
Posterior

- **Lateral position:** A side view with the side of interest placed closest to the Bucky. (A true lateral is 90° from an AP or a PA position).

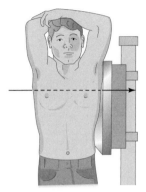

Left lateral projection.

- **Decubitus position:** A horizontal beam is used with the patient lying down. The patient may be in a lateral decubitus position, dorsal decubitus position (patient lying on the back), or a ventral decubitus position (patient is lying on the stomach).

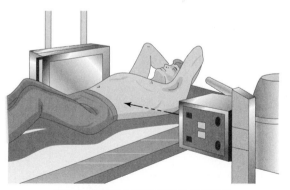

Dorsal decubitus position; lateral projection.

- **Plantar:** Referring to the sole of the foot.
- **Dorsum/dorsal:** Referring to the top of the foot or hand.
- **Palmar (volar):** Referring to the palm of the hand.

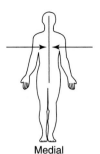

Medial

- **Medial:** Referring to the center of the body.

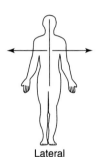

Lateral

- **Lateral:** Referring to away from the center of the body.

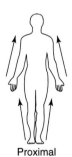

Proximal

- **Proximal:** Towards the trunk of the body.

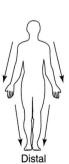

Distal

- **Distal:** Away from the trunk of the body.

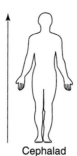

- **Cephalad/cephalic (superior):** Towards the head.

Cephalad

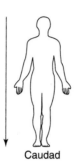

- **Caudad/caudal (inferior):** Towards the feet.

Caudad

- **Ipsilateral:** On the same side.
- **Contralateral:** On the opposite side.
- **Anterior/posterior projection (AP):** This indicates that the x-ray beam enters the anterior surface of the body and exits the posterior surface of the body.

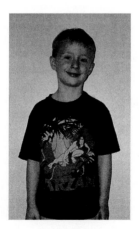

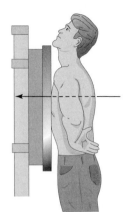

- **Posterior/anterior projection (PA):** This indicates that the x-ray beam enters the posterior surface of the body and exits the anterior surface of the body.

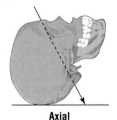

Posteroanterior (PA) projection.

- **Axial projection:** Implies that there is a tube tilt along the long axis of the body (cephalad or caudad).

Axial

- **Transthoracic projection:** A lateral position where the x-ray beam passes through the thorax.
- **Tangential projection:** The x-ray beam skims a body part (sunrise view of the knee, acute flexion of the elbow).

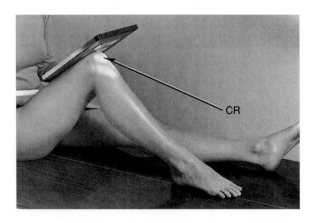

BODY MOVEMENT TERMINOLOGY

- **Abduction:** Movement of a body part away from the trunk of the body.
- **Adduction:** Movement of a body part towards the trunk of the body.

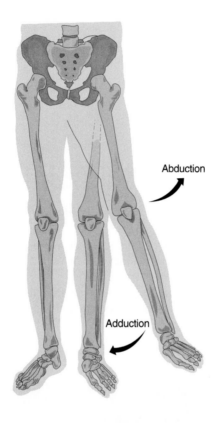

- **Flexion:** Bending of a joint where the angle between the parts is decreased.
- **Extension:** Straightening of a joint where the angle between the parts is increased.

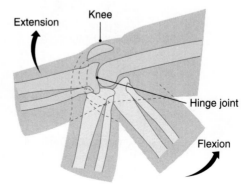

- **Hyperextension:** Implies that the body part was extended beyond the neutral position.
- **Hyperflexion:** Forcible overflexion of a body part.
- **Dorsiflexion:** The top of the foot and toes are pointed upward.
- **Plantar flexion:** The foot and toes are pointed downward.

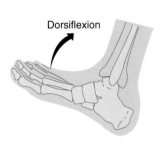

Dorsiflexion

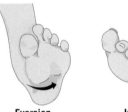
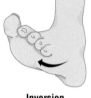

- **Eversion:** Outward movement of the foot and ankle.
- **Inversion:** Inward movement of the foot and ankle.

Eversion   Inversion

- **Radial flexion:** Deviation of the wrist away from the ulnar side (fifth digit) of the forearm, which causes a decrease in the angle between the hand and the radial side of the forearm.
- **Ulnar flexion:** Deviation of the hand away from the radial (thumb) side of the forearm, which causes a decrease in the angle between the hand and ulnar side of the forearm.

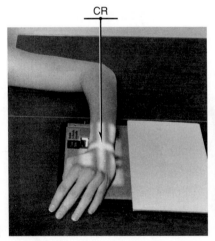
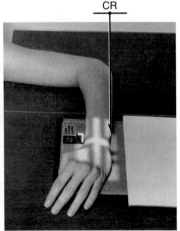

CR   CR

A   B

A. Radial flexion. **B.** Ulnar flexion.

- **Medial rotation (internal rotation):** Rotation of a body part towards the midline of the body.
- **Lateral rotation (external rotation):** Rotation of a body part away from the midline of the body.
- **Pronation:** Rotation of the forearm so that the palm of the hand is flat against the film.
- **Supination:** Rotation of the forearm so that the dorsum of the hand is flat against the film.

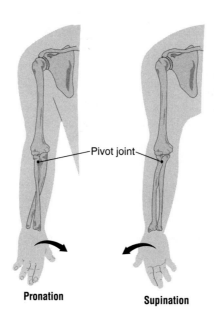

Pronation   Supination

ANATOMIC PLANES

- **Sagittal plane:** Divides the body into right and left parts.
- **Midsagittal plane:** Divides the body into equal right and left parts.
- **Coronal plane (frontal plane):** Divides the body into front and back parts.
- **Midcoronal plane:** Divides the body into equal front and back parts.
- **Transverse plane (horizontal plane):** Divides the body into superior and inferior parts.

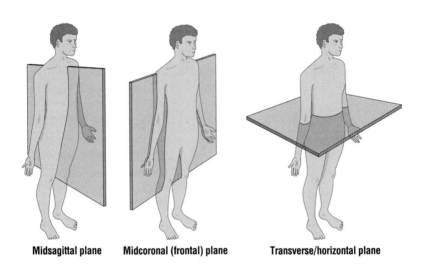

Midsagittal plane   **Midcoronal (frontal) plane**   **Transverse/horizontal plane**

BONY LANDMARKS

Cervical Area

- **C1:** Mastoid tip.
- **C5:** Thyroid cartilage.
- **C7:** Vertebral prominens.

Thoracic Area

- **T2–3:** Level of the superior margin of the scapula.
- **T7:** Level of the inferior angle of the scapula.
- **T10:** Level of the xyphoid tip.

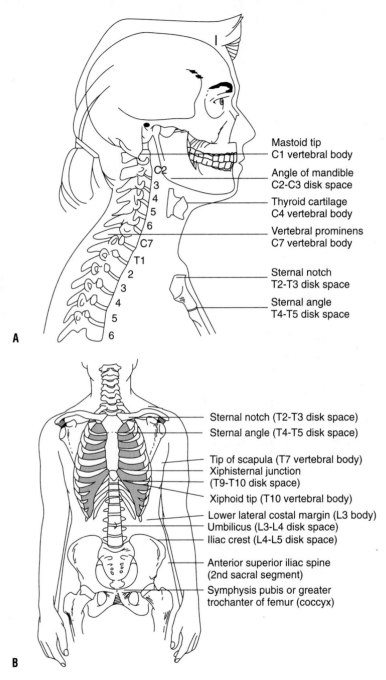

A. Bony landmarks of the neck and spine. **B.** Bony landmarks of the chest and pelvis.

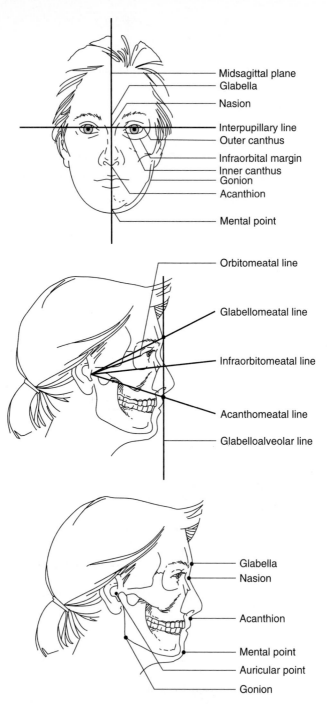

Landmarks of the face and skull.

Lumbar Area
- **L4:** Umbilicus and superior edge of the iliac crest.

Sacrum and Pelvis
- **S1:** Level of the anterior superior iliac spine (ASIS).
- **Coccyx:** Level of the symphysis pubis and greater trochanters.

Head
- **Orbitomeatal line (OML):** Line from outer canthus of the eye to the external auditory meatus (EAM).
- **Glabellomeatal line:** Line from glabella to EAM.
- **Infraorbitomeatal line:** Line from lower margin of the eye to EAM.
- **Acanthiomeatal line:** Line from lower margin of the nose to EAM.

BASIC RULES FOR RADIOGRAPHIC POSITIONING

1. Film Focal Distance (FFD)
The FFD for most procedures is 40 in., except for the following, which are performed at 72 in.:
- Chest x-rays
- Lateral cervical spine films
- Lateral sternum films
- Bilateral acromioclavicular (AC) joints

2. Tube Tilts
- AP projections (AP, RPO, LPO) require cephalic tube tilt.
- PA projections (PA, RAO, LAO) require caudal tube tilt.

Exceptions to rule
- AP coccyx: Caudal tube tilt.
- AP pillar views of cervical spine: Caudal tube tilt.
- Towne's view of skull: Caudal tube tilt.

3. Obliques
- All obliques are midway between an AP or PA and a lateral position (which is usually at 45°).

Exceptions to rule:
- Obliques of thoracic spine.
- Obliques of SI joints.
- Law method of temporomandibular joints (TMJ's).

4. Grids
- Used on all body parts measuring over 12 cm.
- When using a grid, at least 70 kVp should be used to penetrate the grid.

5. Central Ray

- Central ray should be centered to the middle of the anatomy being x-rayed.
- Example: For films of the thoracic spine, T1 through T12, the central ray should be at approximately the T6–7 intervertebral space.

6. Breathing Instructions

All views are performed on suspended expiration except for the following, which are performed on full inspiration:

- Chest x-rays
- Ribs above diaphragm
- Lateral sternum

7. Collimation

- Most states require that three sides of collimation be visible on each film. This demonstrates that only the anatomy being examined is being exposed to radiation.
- Collimate as close to the anatomy as possible without eliminating it from the film.
- Close collimation increases detail on the film (because of absorption of radiation of scatter radiation), but decreases the amount of radiation exposure to the patient.

8. Gonadal Shielding

- Gonadal shielding should be used on all children and on adults of child-bearing age.
- General rule of thumb is that anytime the gonads are within 2 in. of radiation exposure, gonadal shielding should be used unless the shield interferes with the anatomy, causing a repeat exposure.

9. Summary

- These basic rules should be committed to memory as common knowledge and only the factors that do not follow the basic rules (red flags) learned.
- It may be helpful to make a summary sheet following each section with a list of only red flags.

SPINAL RADIOGRAPHY

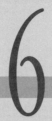

► AP CERVICAL SPINE

- **Anatomy:** C3 through C7 vertebrae, pedicles, spinous processes, intervertebral disc spaces, and uncinate processes.

- **Indication:** The AP view is considered a basic view and should be performed with all cervical spine series. If an abnormality is present, optional views may be indicated. Tomograms or computed tomography (CT) scans may be indicated to rule out fractures or other abnormalities.

- **Film:** 8 × 10 in. or 10 × 12 in. lengthwise with a grid.

- **Tube Tilt:** 15° to 20° cephalad.

- **Film Focal Distance (FFD):** 40 in.

- **Safety:** Collimation should be to the soft tissue of the neck crosswise and slightly less than the length of the film used. Gonadal shielding should be used on all children and on adults of childbearing age.

- **Position:** Place the patient in an upright position with the back against the Bucky and the head slightly extended. The midsagittal plane should be centered to the Bucky. This view may be done with the patient supine.

- **Central Ray:** 15° to 20° cephalad and centered to C5 so the central ray will exit C4.

- **Respiration:** Suspended expiration.

- **Notes:** Elevate the chin slightly to avoid superimposition over C3.

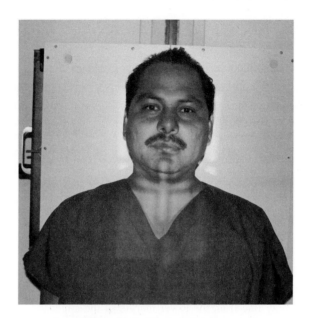

Figure 6–1. AP cervical spine.

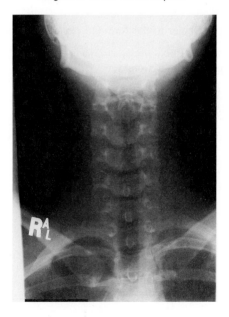

Figure 6–2. AP cervical spine.

▶ AP ODONTOID PROCESS—OPEN MOUTH

- **Anatomy:** Odontoid process, C2 vertebral body, lateral masses of C1.

- **Indication:** The AP odontoid view is a basic view and should be performed with all cervical spine series. If an abnormality is present, optional views may be indicated. Tomograms or CT scans may be indicated to rule out fractures or other abnormalities.

- **Film:** 8 × 10 in. lengthwise with grid.

- **Tube Tilt:** None.

- **FFD:** 40 in.

- **Safety:** Collimate to an area slightly larger than the mouth in an open position. Gonadal shielding should be used on all children and on adults of childbearing age.

- **Position:** Place the patient in an upright position with the back against the Bucky. Instruct the patient to open his or her mouth as wide as possible. An imaginary line from the lower margin of the upper incisors and the base of the skull should be perpendicular to the film. This view may be done with the patient supine.

- **Central Ray:** Perpendicular to the film and centered to the midline of the mouth.

- **Respiration:** Suspended expiration.

- **Notes:**
  1. Ask the patient to remove any dental hardware from the mouth.
  2. Have the patient open his or her mouth after the technician is prepared to take the film. This reduces fatigue and motion on the film.

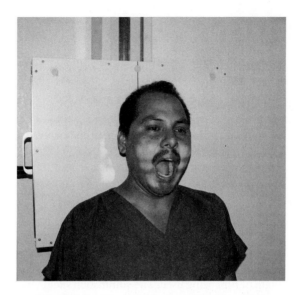

Figure 6–3. AP odontoid process (open mouth).

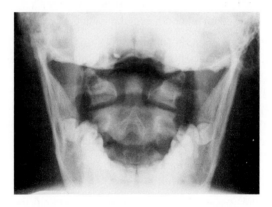

Figure 6–4. AP odontoid process (open mouth).

► NEUTRAL LATERAL CERVICAL SPINE

- **Anatomy:** Intervertebral disc spaces, vertebral bodies, spinous processes, articular pillars, and zygapophyseal joints.

- **Indication:** The lateral view is considered a basic view and is 90° from an AP projection. This view should be performed with all cervical spine series. This is the first film of choice for patients involved in trauma to rule out fracture. If an abnormality is present, optional views may be indicated. A possible fracture may indicate the need for tomograms or CT scans.

- **Film:** 8 × 10 in. or 10 × 12 in. lengthwise with grid.

- **Tube Tilt:** None.

- **FFD:** 72 in.

- **Safety:** Collimate to the soft tissue of the neck crosswise and slightly less than the length of film being used. The collimation should include an area approximately 1 in. above the external auditory meatus (EAM) and 1 in. anterior to the EAM in order to include the sella turcica. Gonadal shielding should be used on all children and on adults of childbearing age.

- **Position:** Place the patient in an upright position with the left side against the Bucky. Instruct the patient to relax and drop the shoulders downward as far as possible. If there is no contraindication, have the patient hold weights of approximately five to ten pounds in each hand, which will aid in pulling the shoulders downward. This view may be done with the patient supine and using a horizontal beam (trauma patients).

- **Central Ray:** Perpendicular to the film and centered to C4.

- **Respiration:** Suspended expiration.

- **Notes:**
  1. Center the cassette 1 to 2 in. above the external auditory meatus (EAM) in order to include the sella turcica, especially on a patient who has complained of frequent headaches.
  2. The 72-in. FFD is used in order to compensate for an increased object film distance (OFD). An increased OFD causes magnification, whereas a 72-in. FFD will decrease magnification.

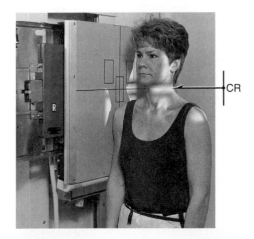

CR

Figure 6–5. Neutral lateral cervical spine.

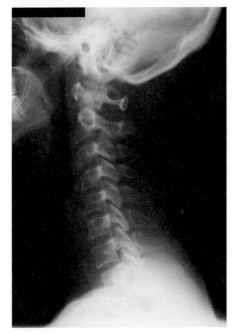

Figure 6–6. Neutral lateral cervical spine.

▶ AP OBLIQUES CERVICAL SPINE (RPO/LPO)

- **Anatomy:** Pedicles and intervertebral foramina furthest from the film.

- **Indication:** This view is recommended when encroachment of the intervertebral foramina is suspected, possibly due to osteophytes, tumors, or other pathology.

- **Film:** 8 × 10 in. or 10 × 12 in. lengthwise with a grid.

- **Tube Tilt:** 15° to 20° cephalad.

- **FFD:** 72 in. (40 in. can be used, but will increase magnification of the intervertebral foramina).

- **Safety:** Collimate to the soft tissue of the neck and slightly less than the length of film being used. Gonadal shielding should be used on all children and on adults of childbearing age.

- **Position:** Place the patient in an upright position with the back against the Bucky. Rotate the patient's body 45° (halfway between an AP and lateral view). The head may be turned towards the film to a near lateral position to avoid superimposition of the mandible and vertebrae and to open up the upper intervertebral foramina. This view may be done with the patient recumbent.

- **Central Ray:** 15° to 20° cephalad and centered to C5 so that the central ray will exit C4.

- **Respiration:** Suspended expiration.

- **Notes:**
  1. Overelevation of the chin will cause superimposition of the base of the skull over C1.
  2. Incorrect tube tilt will obscure the intervertebral disc spaces.
  3. To ensure accurate obliques, place tape on the floor at a 45° angle.

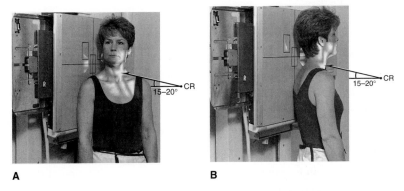

A   **B**

Figure 6–7. **A.** RPO cervical spine. **B.** LPO cervical spine.

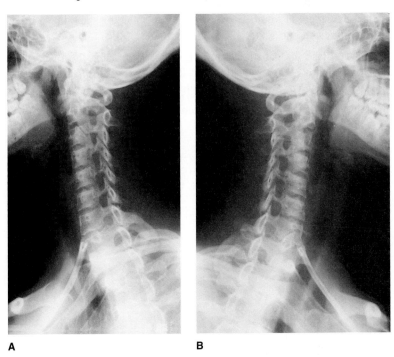

A   **B**

Figure 6–8. **A.** RPO cervical spine. **B.** LPO cervical spine.

▶ PA OBLIQUES CERVICAL SPINE (LAO/RAO)

- **Anatomy:** Pedicles and intervertebral foramina closest to the film.

- **Indication:** This view is recommended when encroachment of the intervertebral foramina is suspected, possibly due to osteophytes, tumors, or other pathology.

- **Film:** 8 × 10 in. or 10 × 12 in. lengthwise with grid.

- **Tube Tilt:** 15° to 20° caudad.

- **FFD:** 72 in. (40 in. can be used but will increase magnification of the intervertebral foramina).

- **Safety:** Collimate to the soft tissue of the neck crosswise and slightly less than the length of film being used. Gonadal shielding should be used on all children and on adults of childbearing age.

- **Position:** Place the patient in an upright position facing the Bucky. The patient's body is then rotated to 45°. The head is turned to a near lateral position. This view may be done with the patient recumbent.

- **Central Ray:** 15° to 20° caudad and centered to C5 so the central ray will exit at C4.

- **Respiration:** Suspended expiration.

- **Notes:** Since anterior obliques visualize the intervertebral foramina closest to the film, less magnification is noted compared to the posterior obliques.

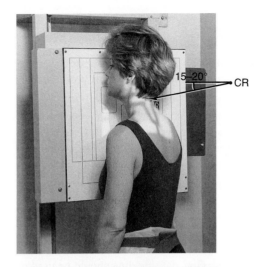

Figure 6–9. RAO cervical spine.

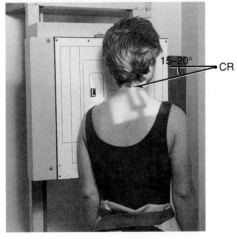

Figure 6–10. LAO cervical spine.

▶ LATERAL HYPERFLEXION CERVICAL SPINE

- **Anatomy:** Vertebral bodies of C1 through C7, spinous processes, intervertebral disc spaces, and zygapophyseal joints. The spinous processes will be separated.

- **Indication:** This view is done in order to demonstrate ligamentous instability and increased or decreased motion in cervical spine trauma. It is contraindicated if a fracture is present. This view may be done 5 to 10 days following trauma to visualize and document the extent of injury.

- **Film:** 10 × 12 in. lengthwise with grid.

- **Tube Tilt:** None.

- **FFD:** 72 in.

- **Safety:** Collimate to the soft tissue of the neck crosswise and slightly less than the length of film being used. Gonadal shielding should be used on all children and on adults of childbearing age.

- **Position:** Place the patient in an upright position with the left side against the Bucky. Instruct the patient to tuck the chin and then flex the neck forward as much as the patient can tolerate.

- **Central Ray:** Perpendicular to the film and centered to the level of C4.

- **Respiration:** Suspended expiration.

- **Notes:**
  1. Make sure the neutral lateral view of the cervical spine shows no fractures or dislocations before attempting this view.
  2. Tucking the chin and then flexing the neck ensures motion in all parts of the cervical spine instead of in the lower cervical spine only.
  3. Make sure the patient is still positioned properly relative to the film when flexing the neck.
  4. Do not attempt to force the patient's neck into flexion past tolerance.

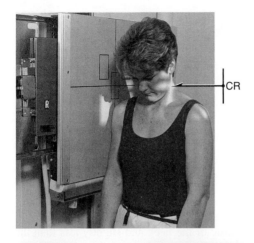

Figure 6–11. Lateral hyperflexion cervical spine.

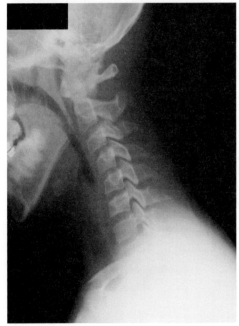

Figure 6–12. Lateral hyperflexion cervical spine.

► LATERAL HYPEREXTENSION CERVICAL SPINE

- **Anatomy:** Vertebral bodies of C1 through C7, intervertebral disc spaces, spinous processes, and zygapophyseal joints. The spinous processes will be close together.

- **Indication:** This view demonstrates ligamentous instability (often seen in whiplash injuries) and increased or decreased motion in cervical spine trauma.

- **Film:** 10 × 12 in. lengthwise with grid.

- **Tube Tilt:** None.

- **FFD:** 72 in.

- **Safety:** Collimate to the soft tissue of the neck and slightly less than the length of film being used. Gonadal shielding should be used on all children and on adults of childbearing age.

- **Position:** Place the patient in an upright position with the left side against the Bucky. Have the patient elevate the chin and lean the head back as far as possible.

- **Central Ray:** Perpendicular to the film and centered to C4.

- **Respiration:** Suspended expiration.

- **Notes:**
  1. Make sure a neutral lateral view of the cervical spine shows no fractures or dislocations before attempting this view.
  2. Make sure the patient is still positioned properly relative to the film upon extension of the neck.

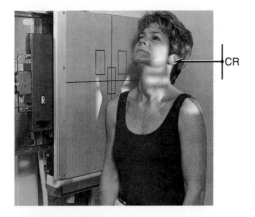

CR

Figure 6–13. Lateral hyperextension cervical spine.

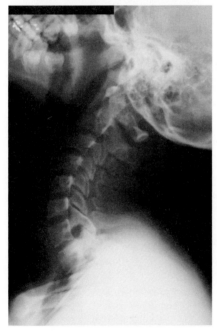

Figure 6–14. Lateral hyperextension cervical spine.

▶ AP CERVICAL SPINE—PILLAR VIEW

- **Anatomy:** Lateral masses of the pillars, articular processes, facets, laminae, and spinous processes free of superimposition of the anterior vertebral body.

- **Indication:** This view should be performed when there is a suspected fracture of the articular pillar. If an abnormality is questionable, then tomograms or CT scans may be indicated.

- **Film:** 8 × 10 in. or 10 × 12 in. lengthwise with grid.

- **Tube Tilt:** 20° to 30° caudad.

- **FFD:** 40 in.

- **Safety:** Collimate to the soft tissue of the neck and slightly less than the length of the film being used. Gonadal shielding should be used on all children and on adults of childbearing age.

- **Position:** Place the patient in the upright position with the back against the Bucky. Instruct the patient to hyperextend his or her head.

- **Central Ray:** 20° to 30° caudad and centered to the upper border of the thyroid cartilage (C5).

- **Respiration:** Suspended expiration.

- **Notes:**
  1. The patient may have to be seated to achieve the required tube tilt.
  2. Do not force the hyperextension past the position that the patient can tolerate.

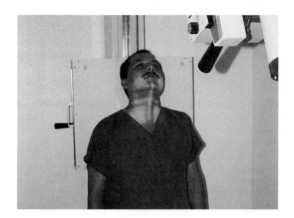

Figure 6–15. A P cervical spine—pillar view.

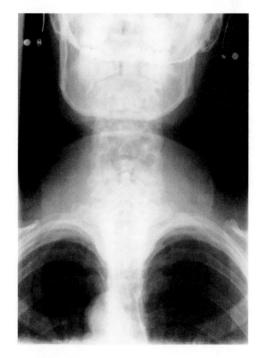

Figure 6–16. AP cervical spine—pillar view.

▶ LATERAL CERVICOTHORACIC SPINE— SWIMMER'S POSITION

- **Anatomy:** Vertebral bodies of the lower cervical and upper thoracic spine, intervertebral disc spaces, spinous processes and the zygapophyseal joints.

- **Indication:** This is an alternative view used to visualize the lower cervical and upper thoracic vertebrae in a lateral position projected between the shadows of the shoulders. This view is used when visualization is impossible in a true lateral projection. Optional views may not be done until all seven cervical vertebrae are seen in a lateral position and fractures are ruled out.

- **Film:** 10 × 12 in. lengthwise with grid.

- **Tube Tilt:** 5° caudad.

- **FFD:** 40 in.

- **Safety:** Collimate to the soft tissue of the cervicothoracic region and slightly less than the length of film being used. Gonadal shielding should be used on all children and on adults of childbearing age.

- **Position:** Place the patient in an upright position with the left side against the Bucky. Have the patient raise the arm closest to the film above the head, flex the elbow, and rest the forearm on the head. The opposite shoulder should be depressed as much as possible. Place the shoulder closest to the film slightly posterior and the opposite shoulder slightly anterior.

- **Central Ray:** 5° caudad and centered to C7-T1 region.

- **Respiration:** Suspended expiration.

- **Notes:**
  1. If the patient is unable to raise his or her left arm above the head, then place the patient in a right lateral position.
  2. This view may also be performed by depressing the arm closest to the film and raising the arm furthest from the film above the patient's head. Use a 5° cephalic tube tilt when performing it in this manner.

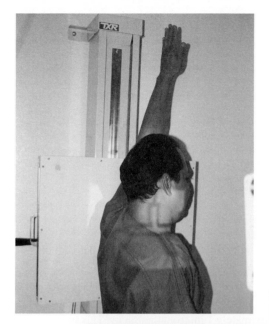

Figure 6–17. Lateral cervicothoracic spine—swimmer's position.

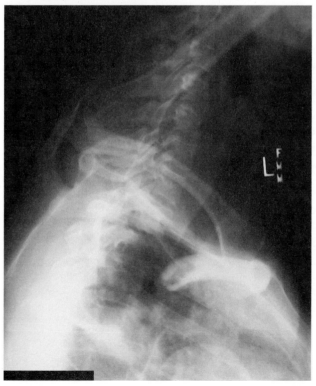

Figure 6–18. Lateral cervicothoracic spine—swimmer's position.

► PA ODONTOID PROCESS—JUDD'S METHOD

- **Anatomy:** C1–C2 in a PA projection with the dens projected through the foramen magnum.

- **Indication:** This is an alternative method used to visualize the odontoid process through the foramen magnum when it is not completely visible on an AP open-mouth odontoid view.

- **Film:** 8 × 10 in. lengthwise with grid.

- **Tube Tilt:** None.

- **FFD:** 40 in.

- **Safety:** Collimate to an area approximately 5 × 5 in. Gonadal shielding should be used on all children and on adults of childbearing age.

- **Position:** Place the patient in an upright position facing the Bucky. Instruct the patient to extend the neck and rest the chin against the Bucky. The tip of the nose should be approximately 1 in. from the Bucky. This view may be done with the patient prone.

- **Central Ray:** Perpendicular to the film and centered to the occiput just posterior to the mastoid processes.

- **Respiration:** Suspended expiration.

- **Notes:** This view may be taken in an AP position with the chin extended to the point that it forms a vertical line with the mastoid processes.

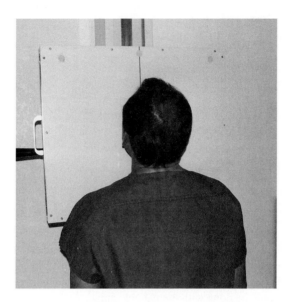

Figure 6–19. PA odontoid process—Judd's method.

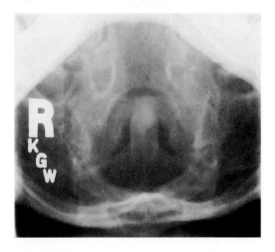

Figure 6–20. PA odontoid process—Judd's method.

▶ AP AXIAL OBLIQUE ODONTOID PROCESS— KASA BACH'S METHOD

- **Anatomy:** Oblique view of C1–C2 with visualization of the dens.

- **Indication:** This is an alternative view used to visualize the odontoid process free of superimposition of the teeth or occiput.

- **Film:** 8 × 10 in. lengthwise with grid.

- **Tube Tilt:** 10° to 15° caudad.

- **FFD:** 40 in.

- **Safety:** Collimate to an area approximately 5 × 5 in. Gonadal shielding should be used on all children and on adults of childbearing age.

- **Position:** Place the patient in an upright position with the back against the Bucky. Instruct the patient to rotate the head 45° away from the side of interest. The infraorbitomeatal line should be perpendicular to the film. This view may be done with the patient supine.

- **Central Ray:** 10° to 15° caudad and centered midway between the external auditory meatus and the lateral canthus of the eye.

- **Respiration:** Suspended expiration.

- **Notes:** This view also visualizes the atlanto-occipital articulations. It may be necessary to modify the head rotation from 35° to 60°.

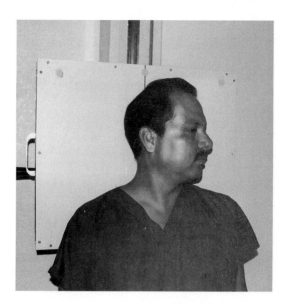

Figure 6–21. AP axial oblique odontoid process—Kasa Bach's method.

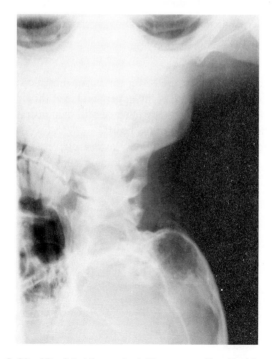

Figure 6–22. AP axial oblique odontoid process—Kasa Bach's method.

▶ AP THORACIC SPINE

- **Anatomy:** Vertebral bodies, pedicles, spinous processes, transverse processes, posterior ribs, costovertebral articulations, and intervertebral disc spaces.

- **Indication:** This is considered a basic view of the thoracic spine and should be performed with all thoracic spine series. If an abnormality is present, then optional views may be indicated. Fractures may be an indication for a CT scan.

- **Film:** 14 × 17 in. or 7 × 17 in. lengthwise with grid.

- **Tube Tilt:** None.

- **FFD:** 40 in.

- **Safety:** Collimate to the width of the spine (approximately 4 in.) crosswise and slightly less than the length of film used. Gonadal shielding should be used on all children and on adults of childbearing age.

- **Position:** Place the patient in an upright position with the back against the Bucky. This view may be done with the patient supine.

- **Central Ray:** Perpendicular to the film and centered to T6.

- **Respiration:** Suspended expiration.

- **Notes:**
  1. A cervicothoracic filter used over the upper thoracic spine obtains a more consistent exposure of the upper and lower thoracic spine.
  2. A diagnostic film of the thoracic spine will demonstrate the thoracic spine through the shadow of the heart.
  3. A thoracic spine film demonstrates the thoracic vertebrae, not the lung fields (so exposure factors for the thoracic spine must be used).

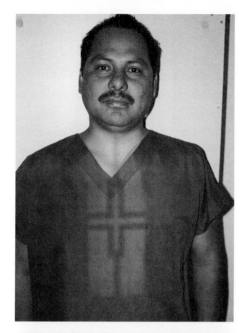

Figure 6–23. AP thoracic spine.

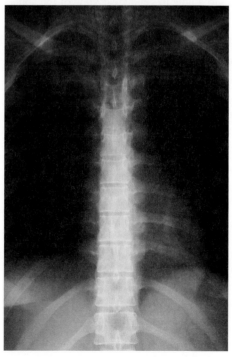

Figure 6–24. AP thoracic spine.

▶ LATERAL THORACIC SPINE

- **Anatomy:** Vertebral bodies, intervertebral foramina, and intervertebral disc spaces.

- **Indication:** This view is considered a basic view of the thoracic spine and should be performed with all thoracic spine series. If the upper thoracic vertebrae are not visible, then a swimmer's view is indicated.

- **Film:** 14 × 17 in. or 7 × 17 in. lengthwise with grid.

- **Tube Tilt:** None.

- **FFD:** 40 in.

- **Safety:** Collimate to the spine crosswise and slightly less than the length of film being used. Gonadal shielding should be used on all children and on adults of childbearing age.

- **Position:** Place the patient in an upright position with the left side against the Bucky. Position the patient's arms above the head or in front of the body, stabilized by holding on to a pole to get a clear view of the spine. This view may be done with the patient recumbent.

- **Central Ray:** Perpendicular to the film and centered at T6.

- **Respiration:** Suspended expiration.

- **Notes:**
  1. If the upper thoracic spine is not visible, perform a swimmer's view.
  2. A breathing technique may be used to blur out ribs and lung markings with motion. Have the patient take shallow breaths. Set the exposure factors with a low mA, 3–4 seconds, and 60–68 kVp.

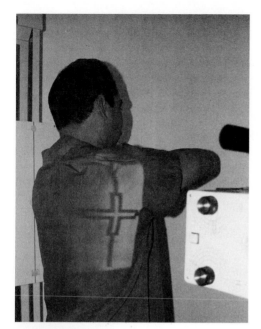

Figure 6–25. Lateral thoracic spine.

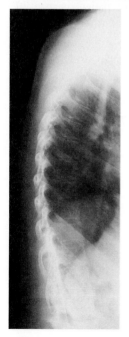

Figure 6–26. Lateral thoracic spine.

► AP/PA OBLIQUES THORACIC SPINE

- **Anatomy:** AP obliques (RPO/LPO) demonstrate the zygapophyseal joints farthest from the film. PA obliques (LAO/RAO) demonstrate the zygapophyseal joints closest to the film.

- **Indication:** Oblique views of the thoracic spine are performed to rule out specific pathology to the zygapophyseal joints.

- **Film:** 14 × 17 in. or 7 × 17 in. lengthwise with grid.

- **Tube Tilt:** None.

- **FFD:** 40 in.

- **Safety:** Collimate to the spine crosswise and slightly less than the length of film being used. Gonadal shielding should be used on all children and on adults of childbearing age.

- **Position:** Place the patient in an upright position with one side against the Bucky. Rotate the patient 20° from a true lateral position. For AP obliques of the thoracic spine, the patient rotates until the back is against the Bucky, whereas on a PA oblique of the thoracic spine, the patient rotates until the chest is against the Bucky. (The patient is in a 70° oblique from an AP position.) This view may be done with the patient recumbent.

- **Central Ray:** Perpendicular to the film and centered to the level T6 and approximately 2 in. lateral to the spine.

- **Respiration:** Suspended expiration.

- **Notes:** Always perform both sides for comparison views.

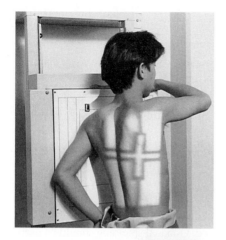

Figure 6–27. LAO thoracic spine.

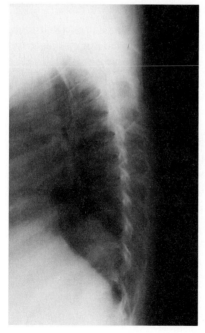

Figure 6–28. LAO thoracic spine.

► AP LUMBAR SPINE

- **Anatomy:** L1 through L5 vertebral bodies, transverse processes, spinous processes, intervertebral disc spaces, laminae, and psoas muscle.
- **Indication:** This is considered a basic view of the lumbar spine and is included with all lumbar spine series. If an abnormality is present, optional views may be indicated.
- **Film:** 14 × 17 in. or 7 × 17 in. lengthwise with a grid.
- **Tube Tilt:** None.
- **FFD:** 40 in.
- **Safety:** Collimate to the spine crosswise (approximately 4 in.) and slightly less than the length of film being used. Gonadal shielding should be used on all patients as long as the anatomy is not obscured.
- **Position:** Place the patient in an upright position with the back against the Bucky. The midsagittal plane should be centered to the Bucky. This view may be done with the patient supine.
- **Central Ray:** Perpendicular to the film and centered to L4.
- **Respiration:** Suspended expiration.
- **Notes:**
  1. Knees may be flexed to place the lumbar spine closest to the Bucky and take the stress off the lumbar spine.
  2. This view may also be performed with the patient in a PA position.

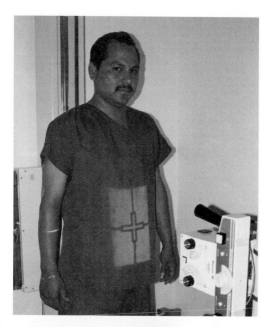

Figure 6–29. AP lumbar spine.

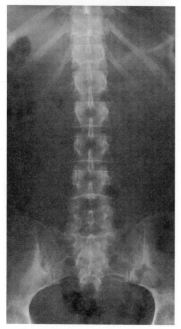

Figure 6–30. AP lumbar spine.

► LATERAL LUMBAR SPINE

- **Anatomy:** Vertebral bodies of L1 through L5, sacrum, intervertebral disc spaces, intervertebral foramina, spinous processes, and pedicles.

- **Indication:** This view is considered a basic view for the lumbar spine and should be done with all lumbar spine series. If an abnormality is present, optional views may be indicated.

- **Film:** 11 × 14 in. or 14 × 17 in. lengthwise with a grid.

- **Tube Tilt:** None.

- **FFD:** 40 in.

- **Safety:** Collimate to the spine crosswise and slightly less than the length of the film being used. Gonadal shielding should be used on all patients as long as the anatomy is not obscured.

- **Position:** Place the patient in an upright position with the left side against the Bucky. This places the patient in a true lateral position. Make sure that the pelvis is not rotated and the arms are raised out of the way. This view may be done with the patient recumbent.

- **Central Ray:** Perpendicular to the film and centered to the level of L4 and approximately 1 in. posterior to the midaxillary line. (L4 is at the level of the iliac crest.) If using 11 × 14 in. film, then the central ray should be at the level of L3.

- **Respiration:** Suspended expiration.

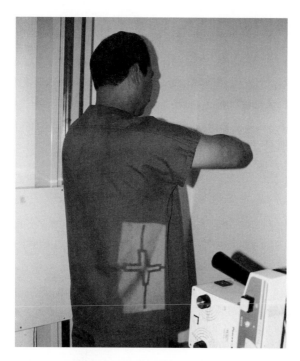

Figure 6–31. Lateral lumbar spine.

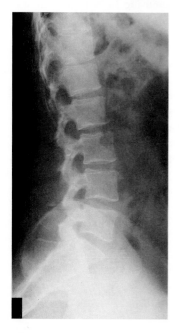

Figure 6–32. Lateral lumbar spine.

► OBLIQUES LUMBAR SPINE (ANTERIOR AND POSTERIOR)

- **Anatomy:** Vertebral bodies, transverse processes, zygapophyseal joints, pedicles, and pars interarticularis.

- **Indication:** Oblique views of the lumbar spine are performed to rule out pars interarticularis fractures.

- **Film:** 11 × 14 in. or 14 × 17 in. lengthwise with a grid.

- **Tube Tilt:** None.

- **FFD:** 40 in.

- **Safety:** Collimate to the spine crosswise and slightly less than the film being used. Gonadal shielding should be used on all patients as long as the anatomy is not obscured.

- **Position:** For AP obliques (RPO/LPO), place the patient in an upright position with the back against the Bucky. Rotate the patient's body 45°. For PA obliques (RAO/LAO), place the patient in an upright position with the abdomen against the Bucky. Rotate the patient's body 45°. These views may be done with the patient recumbent.

- **Central Ray:** If using 11 × 14 in. film, the central ray should be perpendicular to the film and at the level of L3. When using 14 × 17 in. film, the central ray should be perpendicular to the film and at the level of L4 (iliac crest).

- **Respiration:** Suspended expiration.

- **Notes:**
  1. AP obliques (RPO/LPO) demonstrate the side closest to the film, giving less magnification. PA obliques (RAO/LAO) demonstrate the side farthest from the film, creating magnification.
  2. On 45° positioning, a "scotty dog" is visualized.
  3. A fracture of the pars interarticularis will demonstrates a "collar" around the neck of the "scotty dog."

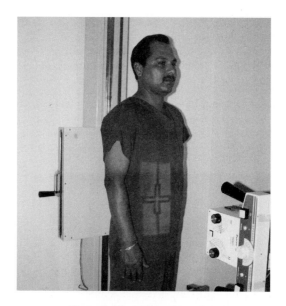

Figure 6–33. LPO lumbar spine.

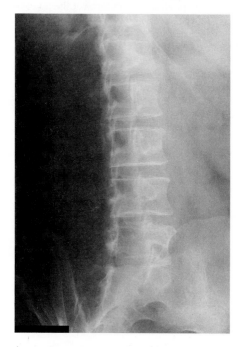

Figure 6–34. LPO lumbar spine.

► AP AXIAL LUMBAR SPINE (L5 SPOT)

- **Anatomy:** L5–S1 lumbosacral joint, L5 vertebral body, upper sacrum, and sacroiliac joints.

- **Indication:** AP L5–S1 spot film is an optional view that is performed to visualize the L5–S1 intervertebral disc space without bony superimposition.

- **Film:** 8 × 10 in. lengthwise with a grid.

- **Tube Tilt:** 30° cephalad for males, 35° cephalad for females.

- **FFD:** 40 in.

- **Safety:** Collimate to a 4 ×4 in. area over the L5–S1 disc space. Gonadal shielding should be used on all patients as long as the anatomy is not obscured.

- **Position:** Place the patient in an upright position with the back against the Bucky. The midsagittal plane should be centered to the film. This view may be done with the patient supine.

- **Central Ray:** 30° to 35° cephalad and centered at the level of the anterior superior iliac spine? (ASIS).

- **Respiration:** Suspended expiration.

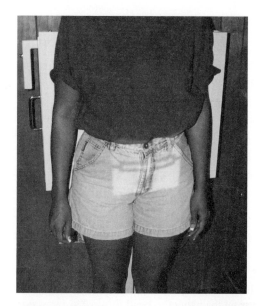

Figure 6–35. AP axial lumbar spine.

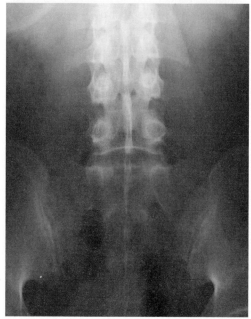

Figure 6–36. AP axial lumbar spine.

▶ LATERAL FLEXION AND EXTENSION LUMBAR SPINE

- **Anatomy:** L1 through L5 vertebral bodies, the sacrum, spinous processes and intervertebral foramina.

- **Indication:** These views are indicated in patients with suspected spinal instability or previous spinal surgery where a fusion has been performed. These views demonstrate the anterior to posterior mobility at the fusion site.

- **Film:** 14 × 17 in. lengthwise with a grid.

- **Tube Tilt:** None.

- **FFD:** 40 in.

- **Safety:** Collimate to the spine crosswise and slightly less than the length of film being used. Gonadal shielding should be used on all patients as long as the anatomy is not obscured.

- **Position:** Place the patient in an upright position with the left side against the Bucky. For flexion, instruct the patient to bend forward as far as possible. For extension, instruct the patient to bend backwards as far as possible. This view may be performed with the patient recumbent.

- **Central Ray:** Perpendicular to the film and centered to the level of L4 (iliac crest).

- **Respiration:** Suspended expiration.

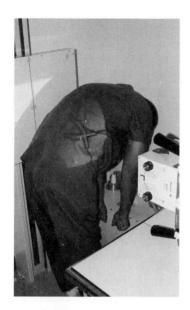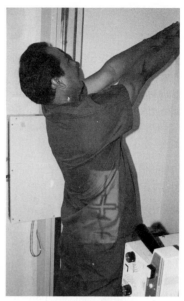

Figure 6–37. A. Lateral flexion lumbar spine. **B.** Lateral extension lumbar spine.

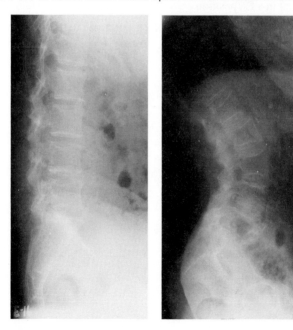

Figure 6–38. A. Lateral flexion lumbar spine. **B.** Lateral extension lumbar spine.

► AP LATERAL BENDING LUMBAR SPINE

- **Anatomy:** Lower and upper lumbar vertebral bodies, intervertebral disc spaces, spinous processes, and pedicles.

- **Indication:** These views are indicated on patients with previous spinal surgery and spinal fusion. These views demonstrate range of motion of the spine at the site of the fusion.

- **Film:** 14 × 17 in. lengthwise with a grid.

- **Tube Tilt:** None.

- **FFD:** 40 in.

- **Safety:** Collimate to the spine crosswise and slightly less than the length of film being used. Gonadal shielding should be used on all patients as long as the anatomy is not obscured.

- **Position:** Place the patient in an upright position with the back against the Bucky. For right lateral bending have the patient bend to the right; for left lateral bending have the patient bend to the left. The midsagittal plane should be centered to the center of the film. This view may be done with the patient in a PA position.

- **Central Ray:** Perpendicular to the film and centered to the level of L4 (iliac crest).

- **Respiration:** Suspended expiration.

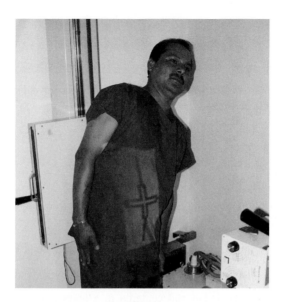

Figure 6–39. AP lateral bending lumbar spine.

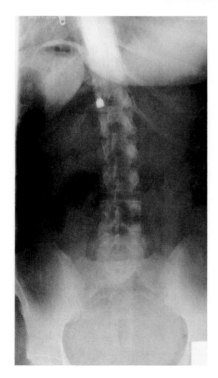

Figure 6–40. AP lateral bending lumbar spine.

► AP SACRUM

- **Anatomy:** L5 vertebral body, sacrum, sacral foramina, and sacroiliac joints.
- **Indication:** This is considered a basic view of the sacrum and should be performed with all sacral series.
- **Film:** 10 × 12 in. lengthwise with a grid.
- **Tube Tilt:** 15° cephalad.
- **FFD:** 40 in.
- **Safety:** Collimate to a size slightly less than the size of film being used. Gonadal shielding should be used on all patients as long as the anatomy is not obscured.
- **Position:** Place the patient in an upright position with the back against the Bucky. The midsagittal plane should be centered to the midline of the film. This view may be done with the patient supine.
- **Central Ray:** 15° cephalad and centered to a point midway between the symphysis pubis and the level of the ASIS.
- **Respiration:** Suspended expiration.

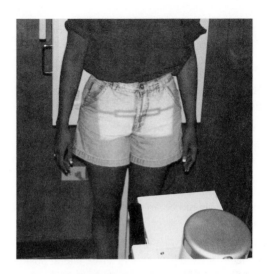

Figure 6–41. AP sacrum.

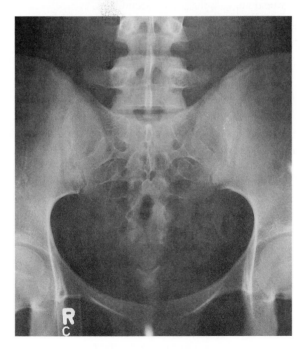

Figure 6–42. AP sacrum.

► LATERAL SACRUM

- **Anatomy:** L5–S1 joint space, sacrum, and coccyx.

- **Indication:** This is considered a basic view of the sacrum and should be performed with all sacral series.

- **Film:** 10 × 12 in. lengthwise with a grid.

- **Tube Tilt:** None.

- **FFD:** 40 in.

- **Safety:** Collimate to an area slightly less than the size of film being used. Gonadal shielding should be used on all patients as long as the anatomy is not obscured.

- **Position:** Place the patient in an upright position with the left side against the Bucky. Make sure the patient is in a true lateral position, without any rotation of the pelvis. The arms should be raised out of the way. This view may be done with the patient recumbent.

- **Central Ray:** Perpendicular to the film and centered to the level of the ASIS and approximately 2 in. anterior to the posterior aspect of the body, halfway between the midaxillary line and the most posterior aspect of the body.

- **Respiration:** Suspended expiration.

- **Notes:**
  1. The lateral view of the sacrum and coccyx are usually taken as one film.
  2. AP projections of the sacrum and coccyx must be taken separately due to different tube tilts and direction of angulation.

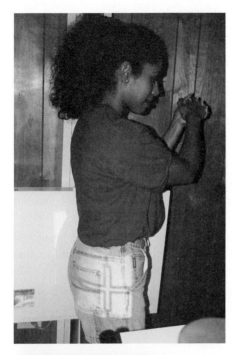

Figure 6–43. Lateral sacrum.

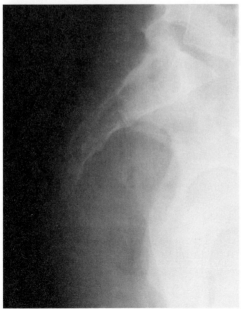

Figure 6–44. Lateral sacrum.

► AP COCCYX

- **Anatomy:** Coccyx and lower sacrum.

- **Indication:** This is considered a basic view and should be performed with all coccygeal series.

- **Film:** 8 × 10 in. lengthwise with a grid.

- **Tube Tilt:** 10° caudad.

- **FFD:** 40 in.

- **Safety:** Collimate to an area approximately 4 × 4 in. over the coccyx. Gonadal shielding should be used on all patients as long as the anatomy is not obscured.

- **Position:** Place the patient in an upright position with the back against the Bucky. The midsagittal plane should be centered to the midline of the film. This view may be done with the patient supine.

- **Central Ray:** 10° caudad and centered approximately 2 in. superior to the symphysis pubis and to the midsagittal plane.

- **Respiration:** Suspended expiration.

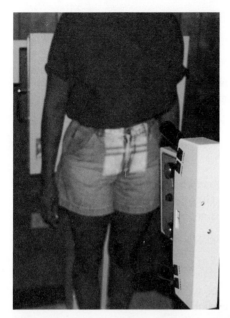

Figure 6–45. AP coccyx.

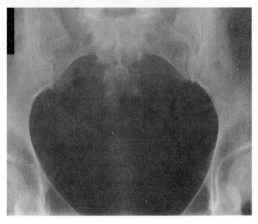

Figure 6–46. AP coccyx.

► LATERAL COCCYX

- **Anatomy:** Coccyx and sacrum.

- **Indication:** This is considered a basic view of the coccyx and should be performed with all coccygeal series.

- **Film:** 8 × 10 in. or 10 × 12 in. lengthwise with a grid.

- **Tube Tilt:** None.

- **FFD:** 40 in.

- **Safety:** Collimate to the sacrum and coccyx crosswise and slightly less than the size of film being used. Gonadal shielding should be used on all patients as long as the anatomy is not obscured.

- **Position:** Place the patient in an upright position with the left side against the Bucky.

- **Central Ray:** Perpendicular to the film and centered to the level of the ASIS and approximately 2 in. anterior to the posterior aspect of the body, midway between the midaxillary line and the most posterior aspect of the body.

- **Respiration:** Suspended expiration.

- **Notes:** The lateral sacrum and coccyx may be performed as one film.

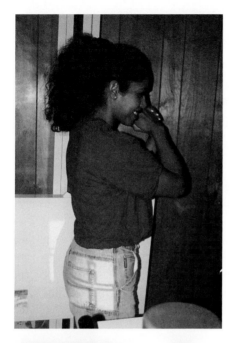

Figure 6–47. Lateral coccyx.

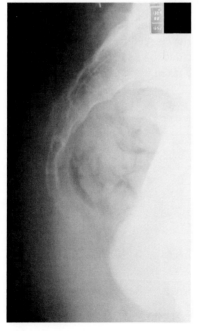

Figure 6–48. Lateral coccyx.

► AP AXIAL SACROILIAC JOINTS

- **Anatomy:** Sacroiliac joints, sacrum, coccyx, and L5–S1 joint space.

- **Indication:** This is considered a basic view of the sacroiliac joints and should be performed with all sacroiliac joint series.

- **Film:** 10 × 12 in. lengthwise with a grid.

- **Tube Tilt:** 30° cephalad for males and 35° cephalad for females.

- **FFD:** 40 in.

- **Safety:** Collimate to an area slightly less than the size of film being used. Gonadal shielding should be used on all patients as long as the anatomy is not obscured.

- **Position:** Place the patient in an upright position with the back against the Bucky. The midsagittal plane should be centered to the film. This view may be done with the patient supine.

- **Central Ray:** 30° to 35° cephalad and centered midway between the ASIS and the symphysis pubis.

- **Respiration:** Suspended expiration.

- **Notes:**
  1. This view may be performed with the patient in a PA position with a 30° to 35° caudad tube tilt. This view is preferred for better visualization of the joint closest to the film due to less magnification.
  2. An AP view of the pelvis may be taken in place of the AP axial projection of the sacroiliac joints.

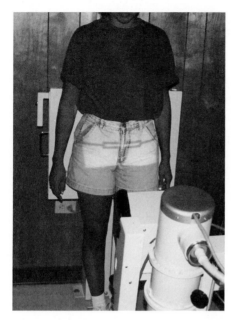

Figure 6–49. AP axial sacroiliac joints.

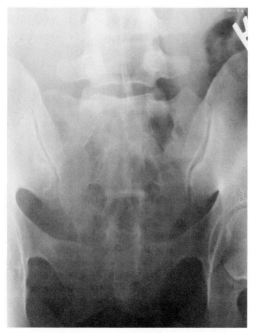

Figure 6–50. AP axial sacroiliac joints.

► OBLIQUE SACROILIAC JOINTS (ANTERIOR AND POSTERIOR)

- **Anatomy:** AP obliques (LPO and RPO) demonstrate the sacroiliac joint farthest from the film. PA obliques (LAO and RAO) demonstrate the sacroiliac joints closest to the film.

- **Indication:** These views are considered basic views and should be performed with all sacroiliac joint series. If abnormalities are present, special imaging may be indicated such as CT scan, MRI, or radionuclide scan.

- **Film:** 8 × 10 or 10 × 12 in. lengthwise with a grid.

- **Tube Tilt:** None.

- **FFD:** 40 in.

- **Safety:** Collimate to an area slightly less than the size of film being used. Gonadal shielding should be used on all patients as long as the anatomy is not obscured.

- **Position:** Place the patient in an upright position. For AP obliques, the patient's back should be against the Bucky and rotated 30° to an oblique position (LPO/RPO). For PA obliques, the patient should be placed with the abdomen and pelvis against the Bucky and rotated approximately 30° into an oblique position (RAO/LAO). These views may be done with the patient recumbent.

- **Central Ray:** Perpendicular to the film and centered 1 in. medial to the ASIS farthest from the film for AP obliques. For PA obliques, the central ray should be perpendicular to the film and centered 1 in. medial to the downside ASIS.

- **Respiration:** Suspended expiration.

- **Notes:** Always x-ray right and left sacroiliac joints for comparison.

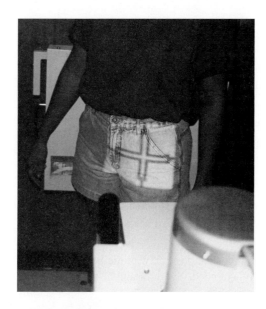

Figure 6–51. RPO sacroiliac joint.

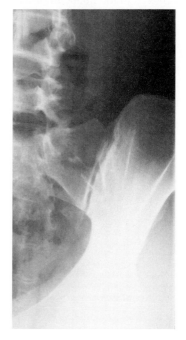

Figure 6–52. RPO sacroiliac joint.

► AP FULL SPINE

- **Anatomy:** Cervical, thoracic, and lumbar vertebral bodies, pedicles, spinous processes, transverse processes, and intervertebral disc spaces.

- **Indication:** This view is sometimes preferred by chiropractors in order to visualize the entire spine as one entity.

- **Film:** 14 × 36 in. lengthwise with a grid.

- **Tube Tilt:** None.

- **FFD:** 72 in.

- **Safety:** Collimate to the spine crosswise and slightly less than the length of the film being used. Gonadal shielding should be used on all patients as long as the anatomy is not obscured.

- **Position:** Place the patient in an upright position with the back against the Bucky and the head slightly extended. The midsagittal plan should be centered to the midpoint of the film.

- **Central Ray:** Perpendicular to the film and centered to the midpoint of the film.

- **Respiration:** Suspended expiration.

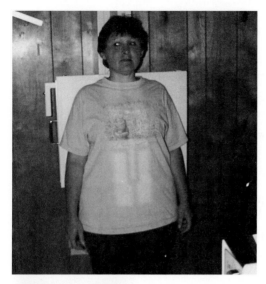

Figure 6–53. AP full spine.

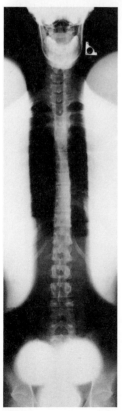

Figure 6–54. AP full spine.

► LATERAL FULL SPINE

- **Anatomy:** Cervical, thoracic, and lumbar vertebral bodies, intervertebral disc spaces, intervertebral foramina, spinous processes, and pedicles.

- **Indication:** This view is sometimes preferred by chiropractors in order to see the entire spine as one entity.

- **Film:** 14 × 36 in. lengthwise with a grid.

- **Tube Tilt:** None.

- **FFD:** 72 in.

- **Safety:** Collimate to the spine crosswise and slightly less than the length of film being used.

- **Position:** Place the patient in an erect position with the left side against the Bucky. Make sure the pelvis is not rotated and the arms are raised out of the way.

- **Central Ray:** Perpendicular to the film and centered to the midpoint of the film.

- **Respiration:** Suspended expiration.

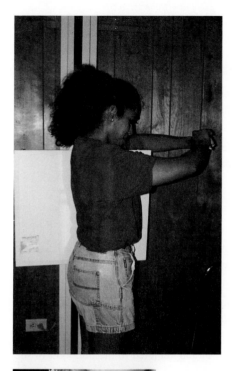

Figure 6–55. Lateral full spine.

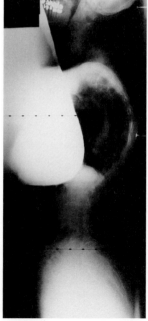

Figure 6–56. Lateral full spine.

► AP AND PA FULL SPINE FOR SCOLIOSIS— FERGUSON'S METHOD

- **Anatomy:** Thoracic and lumbar vertebral bodies in an AP or PA position, pedicles, spinous processes, transverse processes, and intervertebral disc spaces.

- **Indication:** This view is indicated to distinguish between a deforming primary scoliosis and a compensatory scoliosis.

- **Film:** 14 × 17 in. or 14 × 36 in. lengthwise with a grid.

- **Tube Tilt:** None.

- **FFD:** 40 in.

- **Safety:** Collimate to the spine crosswise and slightly less than the length of film being used. Gonadal shielding should be used on all patients as long as the anatomy is not obscured.

- **Position:** Place the patient in an upright position with the abdomen against the Bucky. The midsagittal plane should be centered to the midpoint of the film.

- **Central Ray:** Perpendicular to the film and centered to the midpoint of the film.

- **Respiration:** Suspended expiration.

- **Notes:**
  1. This film may be taken in an AP or PA position.
  2. Once this film is taken, a second radiograph is taken with the foot on the convex side of the curve elevated approximately 3 to 4 in. Place a book or a block underneath the foot to achieve elevation.

UPPER EXTREMITY RADIOGRAPHY

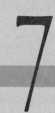

▶ AP SHOULDER WITH INTERNAL ROTATION

- **Anatomy:** Clavicle, acromion, acromioclavicular joint, head of the humerus, glenoid fossa, and lesser tubercle.

- **Indication:** This is considered a basic view of the shoulder that places the head of the shoulder and upper humerus in a lateral position. This view should be performed with all shoulder series, if possible. If an abnormality is present, then optional views may be indicated.

- **Film:** 10 × 12 in. crosswise with a grid.

- **Tube Tilt:** None.

- **FFD:** 40 in.

- **Safety:** Collimate to an area slightly less than the film being used. The film should include proximal and distal ends of the clavicle. Gonadal shielding should be used on all children and on adults of childbearing age.

- **Position:** Place the patient in an upright position with the back against the Bucky. Instruct the patient to internally rotate the arm so that an imaginary line connecting the epicondyles of the elbow is placed perpendicular to the film. This view may be done with the patient supine.

- **Central Ray:** Perpendicular to the film and centered to the coracoid process.

- **Respiration:** Suspended expiration.

- **Notes:** Do not attempt to rotate the arm if a fracture or dislocation is suspected.

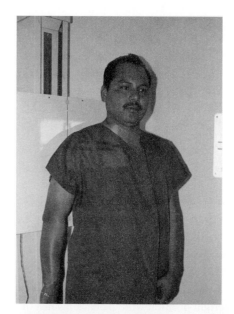

Figure 7–1. AP shoulder with internal rotation.

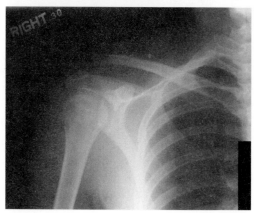

Figure 7–2. AP shoulder with internal rotation.

▶ AP SHOULDER WITH EXTERNAL ROTATION

- **Anatomy:** Clavicle, acromion, acromioclavicular joint, greater tubercle, and glenoid fossa.

- **Indication:** This is a basic view of the shoulder that places the head of the humerus in an AP projection. This view should be performed with all shoulder series. If an abnormality is present, then optional views may be indicated.

- **Film:** 10 × 12 in. crosswise with a grid.

- **Tube Tilt:** None.

- **FFD:** 40 in..

- **Safety:** Collimate to an area slightly less than the film being used. The film should include the proximal and distal ends of the clavicle. Gonadal shielding should be used on all children and on adults of childbearing age.

- **Position:** Place the patient in an upright position with the back against the Bucky. Instruct the patient to externally rotate the arm to a point where an imaginary line between the epicondyles is placed parallel to the film. This view may be done with the patient supine.

- **Central Ray:** Perpendicular to the film and centered to the coracoid process.

- **Respiration:** Suspended expiration.

- **Notes:** Do not attempt to rotate the arm if a fracture or dislocation is suspected.

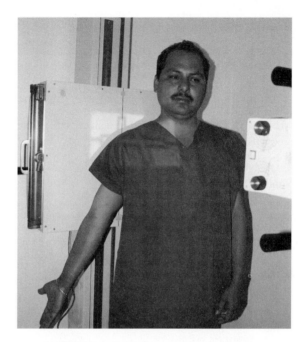

Figure 7–3. AP shoulder with external rotation.

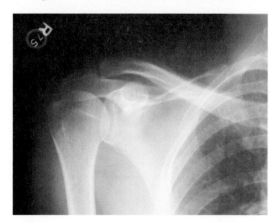

Figure 7–4. AP shoulder with external rotation.

► AP OBLIQUE SHOULDER (RPO/LPO)— GLENOID FOSSA VIEW

- **Anatomy:** Acromion, clavicle, coracoid process, head of the humerus, glenoid fossa, and scapulohumeral joint.

- **Indication:** This is an optional view that visualizes the glenoid fossa in profile and opens the scapulohumeral joint space.

- **Film:** 10 × 12 in. crosswise or lengthwise with a grid.

- **Tube Tilt:** None.

- **FFD:** 40 in.

- **Safety:** Collimate to an area slightly less than the film being used. Gonadal shielding should be used on all children and on adults of childbearing age.

- **Position:** Place the patient in an upright position with the back against the Bucky. Rotate the patient's body 45° towards the affected side (halfway between an AP and lateral position). This view may be done with the patient supine.

- **Central Ray:** Perpendicular to the film and centered to the coracoid process.

- **Respiration:** Suspended expiration.

- **Notes:** This view may be performed with internal and external rotation.

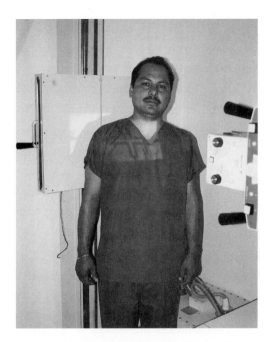

Figure 7–5. RPO shoulder—glenoid fossa view.

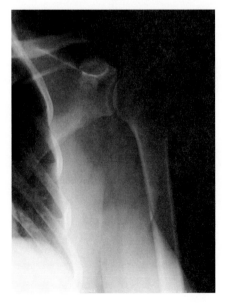

Figure 7–6. RPO shoulder—glenoid fossa view.

▶ TRANSTHORACIC LATERAL SHOULDER

- **Anatomy:** Head of the humerus through the thoracic cavity.

- **Indication:** This view is considered a trauma view and should be performed when a fracture or dislocation of the shoulder is suspected.

- **Film:** 10 × 12 in. lengthwise with a grid.

- **Tube Tilt:** None.

- **FFD:** 40 in.

- **Safety:** Collimate to an area slightly less than the film being used. Gonadal shielding should be used on all children and on adults of childbearing age.

- **Position:** Place the patient in an upright position with the affected side against the Bucky in a true lateral position. The unaffected arm should be placed above the patient's head. This view may be done with the patient supine and using a horizontal beam.

- **Central Ray:** Perpendicular to the film and directed through the thoracic cavity at the level of the neck of the humerus of the affected shoulder.

- **Respiration:** Suspended expiration.

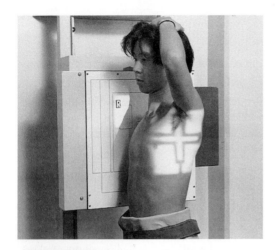

Figure 7–7. Transthoracic lateral shoulder.

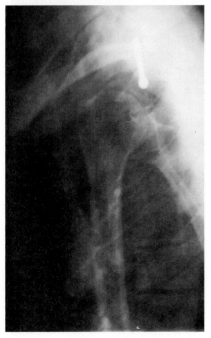

Figure 7–8. Transthoracic lateral shoulder.

▶ PA OBLIQUE SHOULDER (RAO/LAO)—Y VIEW

- **Anatomy:** Clavicle, coracoid process, humerus, and scapula in a lateral projection.

- **Indication:** This view is considered an optional view and should be performed when a fracture or dislocation of the humerus is suspected. This view demonstrates the relationship between the humeral head and the glenoid fossa.

- **Film:** 10 × 12 in. lengthwise with a grid.

- **Tube Tilt:** None.

- **FFD:** 40 in.

- **Safety:** Collimate to an area slightly less than the size of film being used. Gonadal shielding should be used on all children and on adults of childbearing age.

- **Position:** Place the patient in an upright position with the chest against the Bucky. Rotate the patient's body 45° to 60° with the affected side against the film. (Palpate the scapula and place it in a true lateral position.) This view may be done with the patient recumbent.

- **Central Ray:** Perpendicular to the film and centered to the glenohumeral joint.

- **Respiration:** Suspended expiration.

- **Notes:**
  1. When the patient is positioned correctly, the lateral profile of the scapula will form a "Y."
  2. If no dislocation is present, the humeral head will be superimposed over the base of the "Y."

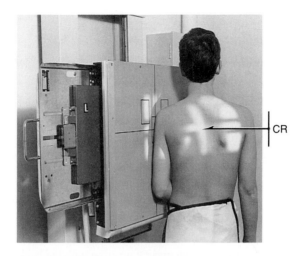

Figure 7–9. PA oblique shoulder—Y-view.

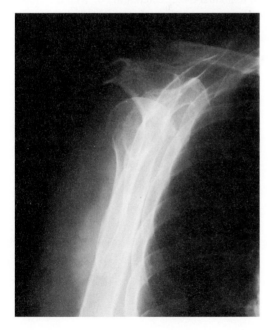

Figure 7–10. PA oblique shoulder—Y-view.

▶ ABDUCTION SHOULDER—BABY ARM VIEW

- **Anatomy:** Humerus, clavicle, acromion, acromioclavicular joint, and coracoid process.

- **Indication:** This is an optional view of the shoulder and should be performed to evaluate the acromion and coracoid process.

- **Film:** 10 × 12 in. crosswise with a grid.

- **Tube Tilt:** None.

- **FFD:** 40 in.

- **Safety:** Collimate to an area slightly less than the film being used. Gonadal shielding should be used on all children and on adults of childbearing age.

- **Position:** Place the patient in an upright position with the back against the Bucky. Instruct the patient to abduct the affected arm 90° with the elbow flexed 90°. This view may be done with the patient supine.

- **Central Ray:** Perpendicular to the film and centered to the coracoid process.

- **Respiration:** Suspended expiration.

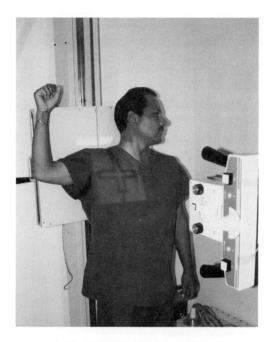

Figure 7–11. Abduction shoulder—baby arm view.

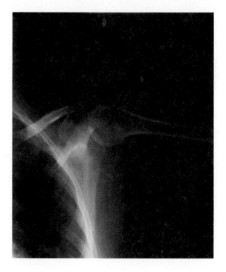

Figure 7–12. Abduction shoulder—baby arm view.

► INFEROSUPERIOR AXIAL SHOULDER

- **Anatomy:** The glenohumeral joint, coracoid process, acromion process, and neck of humerus.

- **Indication:** This in an optional view that is used to rule out fracture and/or dislocation of the humeral head.

- **Film:** 8 × 10 in. or 10 × 12 in. crosswise with a grid.

- **Tube Tilt:** None.

- **FFD:** 40 in.

- **Safety:** Collimate to the soft tissue of the shoulder. Gonadal shielding should be used on all children and on adults of childbearing age.

- **Position:** Place the patient in a supine position with the shoulder abducted to 90°. Externally rotate the patient's arm.

- **Central Ray:** A cassette should be placed against the superior aspect of the shoulder with the central ray directed horizontally and medially through the axilla.

- **Respiration:** Suspended expiration.

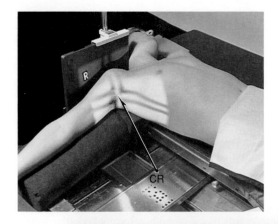

Figure 7–13. Inferosuperior axial shoulder.

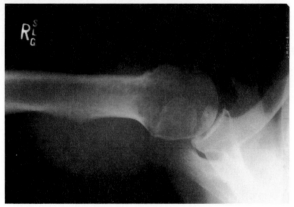

Figure 7–14. Inferosuperior axial shoulder.

► AP ACROMIOCLAVICULAR JOINTS WITHOUT AND WITH WEIGHTS

- **Anatomy:** Acromion, clavicle, acromioclavicular joint, and head of the humerus.

- **Indication:** These views are performed and compared with each other to rule out a separation of the AC joint.

- **Film:** 14 × 17 in. crosswise with a grid.

- **Tube Tilt:** None.

- **FFD:** 72 in.

- **Safety:** Collimate to include soft tissue of both acromioclavicular joints. Gonadal shielding should be used on all children and on adults of child-bearing age.

- **Position:** Place the patient in an upright position with the back against the Bucky. The shoulder should be in a neutral position. A second view is then taken in the same position, with the patient holding a 5-lb. weight in each hand.

- **Central Ray:** Perpendicular to the film and midway between the two acromioclavicular joints (approximately 1 in. above the jugular notch).

- **Respiration:** Suspended expiration.

- **Notes:**
  1. Always perform bilateral acromioclavicular joints to compare one side to the other.
  2. Always perform with and without weights.

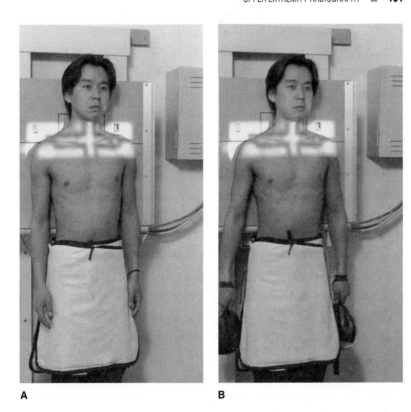

A **B**

Figure 7–15. A. AP acromioclavicular joints without weights. **B.** AP acromioclavicular joints with weights.

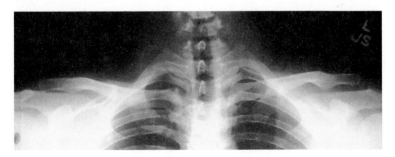

Figure 7–16. AP acromioclavicular joints with weights.

► AP/PA CLAVICLE

- **Anatomy:** Clavicle, acromioclavicular joint, and sternoclavicular joint.

- **Indication:** This is considered a basic view of the clavicle and should be performed with all clavicle series.

- **Film:** 10 × 12 in. crosswise with a grid.

- **Tube Tilt:** None.

- **FFD:** 40 in.

- **Safety:** Collimate to include the proximal and distal ends of the clavicle. Gonadal shielding should be used on all children and on adults of child-bearing age.

- **Position:** *AP:* Place the patient in an upright position with the back against the Bucky; center the clavicle to the middle of the film. *PA:* Place the patient in an upright position with the chest against the Bucky; center the clavicle to the middle of the film. These views may be done with the patient recumbent.

- **Central Ray:** Perpendicular to the film and centered to the midclavicular region.

- **Respiration:** Suspended expiration.

- **Notes:** The PA view of the clavicle demonstrates less magnification due to the fact that it places the clavicle closer to the film.

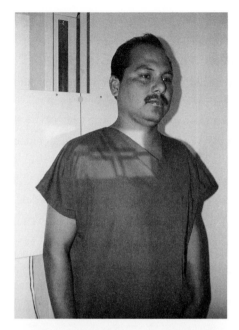

Figure 7–17. AP clavicle.

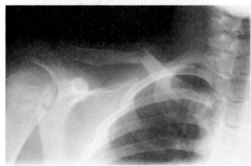

Figure 7–18. AP clavicle.

▶ AP/PA AXIAL CLAVICLE

- **Anatomy:** Clavicle, acromioclavicular joint, and sternoclavicular joint.

- **Indication:** This view is considered a basic view of the clavicle and should be performed with all clavicle series.

- **Film:** 10 × 12 in. crosswise with a grid.

- **Tube Tilt:** 15° to 20° cephalad for the AP view and 15° to 20° caudad for the PA view.

- **FFD:** 40 in.

- **Safety:** Collimate to include the proximal and distal ends of the clavicle. Gonadal shielding should be used on all children and on adults of child-bearing age.

- **Position:** *AP:* Place the patient in an upright position with the back against the Bucky; center the clavicle to the center of the film. *PA:* Place the patient in an upright position with the chest against the Bucky; center the clavicle to the center of the film. This view may be done with the patient recumbent.

- **Central Ray:** *AP:* The central ray is 15° to 20° cephalad and centered to the midclavicular region. *PA:* The central ray is 15° to 20° caudad and centered to the midclavicular region.

- **Respiration:** Suspended expiration.

- **Notes:** AP axial projection projects the clavicle above the apices of the lung, avoiding superimposition.

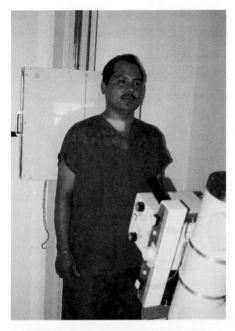

Figure 7–19. AP axial clavicle.

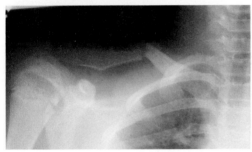

Figure 7–20. AP axial clavicle.

▶ AP SCAPULA

- **Anatomy:** Scapula, coracoid process, acromion, clavicle, glenoid fossa, and head of the humerus.

- **Indication:** This is considered a basic view of the scapula and should be performed with all scapular series.

- **Film:** 10 × 12 in. lengthwise with a grid.

- **Tube Tilt:** None.

- **FFD:** 40 in.

- **Safety:** Collimate to an area slightly less than the film being used. Gonadal shielding should be used on all children and on adults of childbearing age.

- **Position:** Place the patient in an upright position with the back against the Bucky. Instruct the patient to abduct the arm to 90° and flex the elbow to 90°. This view may be done with the patient supine.

- **Central Ray:** Perpendicular to the film and centered to the midscapular region (approximately 2 in. inferior to the coracoid process).

- **Respiration:** Suspended expiration.

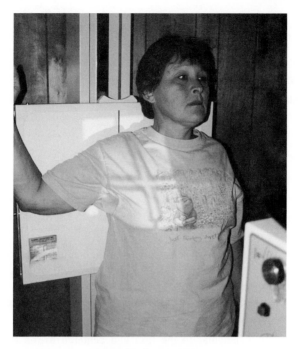

Figure 7–21. AP scapula.

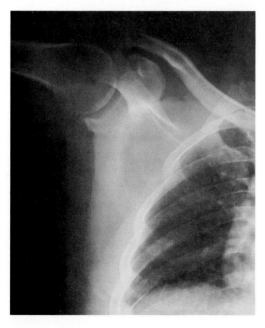

Figure 7–22. AP scapula.

► LATERAL SCAPULA

- **Anatomy:** Scapula, acromion, spine of the scapula, and head of the humerus.

- **Indication:** This view is considered a basic view of the scapula and should be performed with all scapular series.

- **Film:** 10 × 12 in. lengthwise with a grid.

- **Tube Tilt:** None.

- **FFD:** 40 in.

- **Safety:** Collimate to an area slightly less than the film being used. Gonadal shielding should be used on all children and on adults of childbearing age.

- **Position:** Place the patient in an upright position facing the Bucky in an anterior oblique position with the affected side closest to the Bucky. Palpate the border of the scapula and rotate the patient to a point where the scapula is in a true lateral position. This view may be done with the patient recumbent.

- **Central Ray:** Perpendicular to the film and centered to the midscapular region.

- **Respiration:** Suspended expiration.

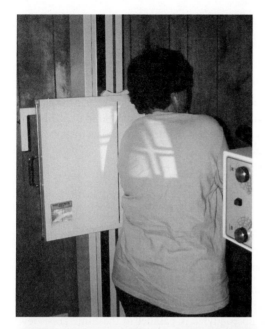

Figure 7–23. Lateral scapula.

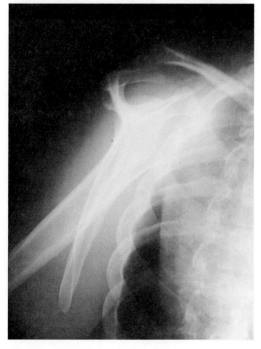

Figure 7–24. Lateral scapula.

▶ AP HUMERUS

- **Anatomy:** Humerus, glenoid fossa, greater tubercle, lesser tubercle, head of the humerus, lateral epicondyle, and medial epicondyle.

- **Indication:** This is considered a basic view of the humerus and should be performed with all humeral series. If the patient is unable to maintain the position required for this view, then a neutral AP and a transthoracic lateral view may be indicated.

- **Film:** 14 × 17 in. lengthwise without a grid.

- **Tube Tilt:** None.

- **FFD:** 40 in.

- **Safety:** Collimate to the soft tissue of the humerus crosswise and include the shoulder and elbow joint lengthwise. Gonadal shielding should be used on all children and on adults of childbearing age.

- **Position:** Place the patient in an upright position with the back against the Bucky. Center the humerus to the film. Supinate the hand so that an imaginary line connecting the epicondyles is parallel to the film. This view may be done with the patient supine.

- **Central Ray:** Perpendicular to the film and centered to the midhumerus.

- **Respiration:** Suspended expiration.

- **Notes:** This view may be done using an extremity cassette.

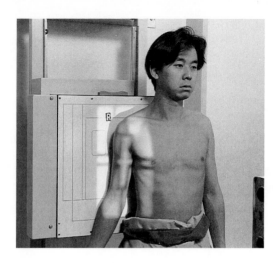

Figure 7–25. AP humerus.

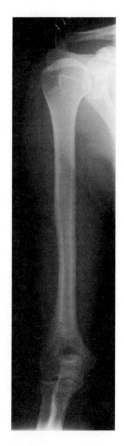

Figure 7–26. AP humerus.

► LATERAL HUMERUS

- **Anatomy:** Humerus, head of the humerus, greater tubercle, lesser tubercle, and medial and lateral epicondyles superimposed.

- **Indication:** This is considered a basic view of the humerus and should be performed with all humeral series. If the patient is unable to maintain the position required to perform this view, then a transthoracic lateral view may be indicated.

- **Film:** 14 × 17 in. lengthwise without a grid.

- **Tube Tilt:** None.

- **FFD:** 40 in.

- **Safety:** Collimate to the soft tissue of the humerus crosswise and include the shoulder and elbow joint lengthwise. Gonadal shielding should be used on all children and on adults of childbearing age.

- **Position:** Place the patient in an upright position with the back against the Bucky. The arm should be placed so that the imaginary line between the medial and lateral epicondyles is perpendicular to the film. This view may be done with the patient supine.

- **Central Ray:** Perpendicular to the film and centered to the midhumerus.

- **Respiration:** Suspended expiration.

- **Notes:** This view may be performed with the patient placed in an anterior oblique with the affected arm against the film. Again, the imaginary line connecting the two epicondyles should be placed perpendicular to the film.

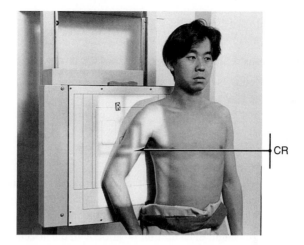

CR

Figure 7–27. Lateral humerus.

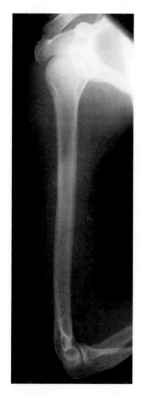

Figure 7–28. Lateral humerus.

▶ TRANSTHORACIC LATERAL HUMERUS

- **Anatomy:** Humerus superimposed with the thoracic cavity.

- **Indication:** This view is indicated when a fracture is suspected and the patient is unable to move the arm.

- **Film:** 14 × 17 in. lengthwise without a grid.

- **Tube Tilt:** None.

- **FFD:** 40 in.

- **Safety:** Collimate to the soft tissue of the humerus crosswise and include the shoulder and elbow joint lengthwise. Gonadal shielding should be used on all children and on adults of childbearing age.

- **Position:** Place the patient in an upright position with the affected humerus against the Bucky. Move the unaffected arm above the patient's head. This places the patient in a true lateral position.

- **Central Ray:** Perpendicular to the film and centered to the midhumeral region through the thoracic cavity.

- **Respiration:** Suspended expiration.

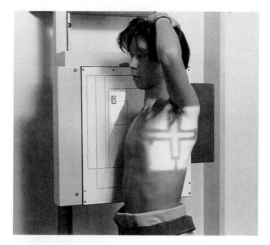

Figure 7–29. Transthoracic lateral humerus.

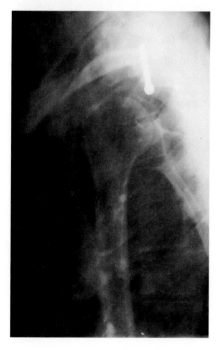

Figure 7–30. Transthoracic lateral humerus.

▶ AP ELBOW

- **Anatomy:** Distal humerus, medial and lateral epicondyles, capitulum, trochlea, proximal radius, olecranon process, and proximal ulna.

- **Indication:** This is a basic view and should be performed with all elbow series. If an abnormality is present, then optional views may be indicated.

- **Film:** 10 × 12 in. crosswise without a grid. The film may be divided in half to include two views.

- **Tube Tilt:** None.

- **FFD:** 40 in.

- **Safety:** Collimate to the soft tissue of the elbow. Gonadal shielding should be used on all children and on adults of childbearing age.

- **Position:** Place the patient in a seated position at a table with the arm placed in the anatomical position. An imaginary line between the two epicondyles should be placed parallel to the film.

- **Central Ray:** Perpendicular to the film and directed to the midelbow joint.

- **Respiration:** Suspended expiration.

- **Notes:** The humerus, elbow, and forearm should all be in the same plane.

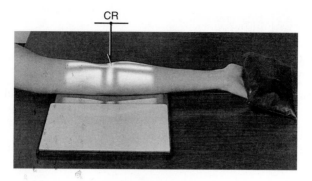

Figure 7–31. AP elbow.

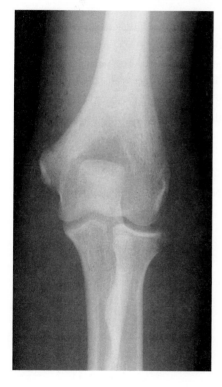

Figure 7–32. AP elbow.

► LATERAL ELBOW

- **Anatomy:** Epicondyles, olecranon process, trochlear notch, radial head, and anterior fat pad.
- **Indication:** This is considered a basic view of the elbow and should be performed with all elbow series. If an abnormality is present, then optional views may be indicated.
- **Film:** 10 × 12 in. crosswise without a grid. The film may be divided in half to include two views.
- **Tube Tilt:** None.
- **FFD:** 40 in.
- **Safety:** Collimate to the soft tissue of the elbow. Gonadal shielding should be used on all children and on adults of childbearing age.
- **Position:** Place the patient in a seated position at a table with the elbow placed in a true lateral position. This is achieved by flexing the elbow to 90° with the thumb pointed towards the ceiling.
- **Central Ray:** Perpendicular to the film and centered to the midelbow joint.
- **Respiration:** Suspended expiration.
- **Notes:**
  1. The humerus, elbow, and forearm should be in the same plane.
  2. Make sure that the patient does not pronate the hand before starting the x-ray.

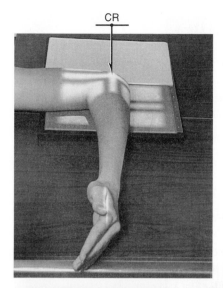

Figure 7–33. Lateral elbow.

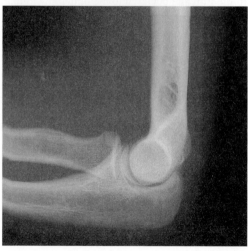

Figure 7–34. Lateral elbow.

► INTERNAL OBLIQUE ELBOW

- **Anatomy:** Olecranon process, coranoid process, radial head, trochlea, and medial epicondyle.

- **Indication:** This view is an optional view and should be performed when a fracture of the olecranon process is suspected.

- **Film:** 10 × 12 in. crosswise without a grid. The film may be divided in half to include two views.

- **Tube Tilt:** None.

- **FFD:** 40 in.

- **Safety:** Collimate to the soft tissue of the elbow. Gonadal shielding should be used on all children and on adults of childbearing age.

- **Position:** Place the patient in a seated position at a table with the arm placed in the anatomic position. Instruct the patient to pronate the hand.

- **Central Ray:** Perpendicular to the film and centered to the midelbow joint.

- **Respiration:** Suspended expiration.

- **Notes:** The humerus, elbow, and forearm should be in the same plane.

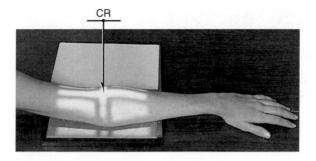

Figure 7–35. Internal oblique elbow.

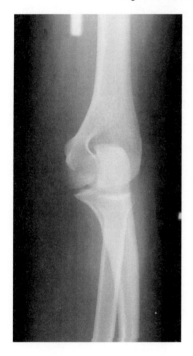

Figure 7–36. Internal oblique elbow.

▶ EXTERNAL OBLIQUE ELBOW

- **Anatomy:** Lateral epicondyle, capitulum, radial head, neck, and tubercle.

- **Indication:** This is an optional view of the elbow that is indicated when a fracture of the radial head neck is suspected.

- **Film:** 10 × 12 in. crosswise without a grid. The film may be divided in half to include two views.

- **Tube Tilt:** None.

- **FFD:** 40 in.

- **Safety:** Collimate to the soft tissue of the elbow. Gonadal shielding should be used on all children and on adults of childbearing age.

- **Position:** Place the patient in a seated position at a table with the arm placed in the anatomical position. Instruct the patient to externally rotate the elbow to a 45° angle.

- **Central Ray:** Perpendicular to the film and centered to the midelbow joint.

- **Respiration:** Suspended expiration.

- **Notes:** Make sure the humerus, elbow, and forearm are in the same plane.

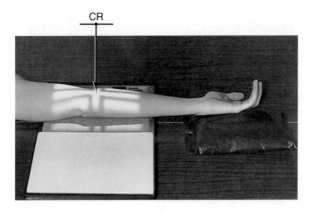

Figure 7–37. External oblique elbow.

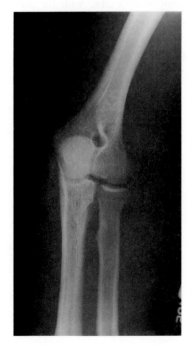

Figure 7–38. External oblique elbow.

► ACUTE FLEXION ELBOW—TANGENTIAL VIEW

- **Anatomy:** Olecranon process, trochlea, capitulum, medial epicondyle, and radial head.

- **Indication:** This is an optional view of the elbow that is indicated when a fracture or dislocation of the olecranon process is suspected.

- **Film:** 8 × 10 in. without a grid.

- **Tube Tilt:** None.

- **FFD:** 40 in.

- **Safety:** Collimate to the soft tissue of the elbow. Gonadal shielding should be used on all children and on adults of childbearing age.

- **Position:** Place the patient in a seated position at a table with the arm placed in the anatomical position. Instruct the patient to flex the elbow as much as possible.

- **Central Ray:** Perpendicular to the film and centered approximately 2 in. superior to the olecranon process.

- **Respiration:** Suspended expiration.

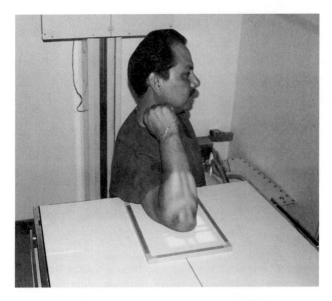

Figure 7–39. Acute flexion elbow—tangential view.

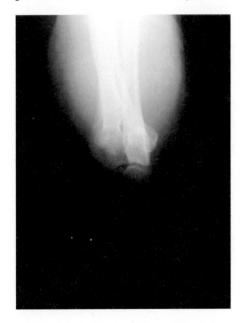

Figure 7–40. Acute flexion elbow—tangential view.

▶ AP FOREARM

- **Anatomy:** Radial and ulnar shaft, radial head, medial and lateral epicondyles, and radial styloid process.

- **Indication:** This is a basic view and should be performed with all forearm series.

- **Film:** 11 × 14 in. crosswise without a grid. The film should be divided in half to include two views.

- **Tube Tilt:** None.

- **FFD:** 40 in.

- **Safety:** Collimate to the soft tissue of the forearm crosswise and include the elbow and wrist joint lengthwise. Gonadal shielding should be used on all children and on adults of childbearing age.

- **Position:** Place the patient in a seated position at a table with the forearm placed in the anatomic position. An imaginary line between the two condyles should be placed parallel to the film.

- **Central Ray:** Perpendicular to the film and centered to the midforearm region.

- **Respiration:** Suspended expiration.

- **Notes:** The humerus, elbow, and forearm should be placed in the same plane.

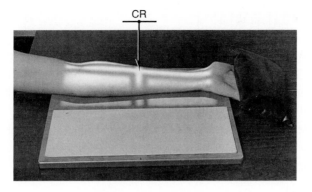

Figure 7–41. AP forearm.

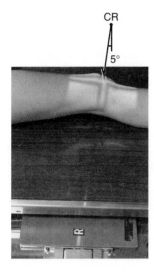

Figure 7–42. AP forearm.

► LATERAL FOREARM

- **Anatomy:** Radial and ulnar shafts, radial head, coronoid process, epicondyles, olecranon process, and ulnar styloid process.

- **Indication:** This is considered a basic view of the forearm and should be performed with all forearm series.

- **Film:** 11 × 14 in. crosswise without a grid. The film should be divided in half to include two views.

- **Tube Tilt:** None.

- **FFD:** 40 in.

- **Safety:** Collimate to the soft tissue of the forearm crosswise and include the elbow and wrist joint lengthwise. Gonadal shielding should be used on all children and on adults of childbearing age.

- **Position:** Place the patient in a seated position at a table with the elbow flexed to 90°. This places the forearm in a true lateral position. Instruct the patient to point the thumb towards the ceiling.

- **Central Ray:** Perpendicular to the film and centered to the midforearm region.

- **Respiration:** Suspended expiration.

- **Notes:** The humerus, elbow, and forearm should be in the same plane.

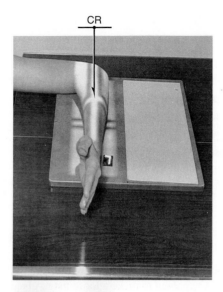

Figure 7–43. Lateral forearm.

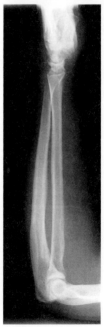

Figure 7–44. Lateral forearm.

▶ PA WRIST

- **Anatomy:** Ulnar and radial styloid processes, scaphoid, lunate, triquetrium, pisiform, trapezium, trapezoid, capitate, and hamate.

- **Indication:** This is considered a basic view of the wrist and should be performed with all wrist series. If an abnormality is present, then optional views may be indicated.

- **Film:** 8 × 10 in. or 10 × 12 in. crosswise without a grid. The film should be divided into half or thirds to include more than one view.

- **Tube Tilt:** None.

- **FFD:** 40 in.

- **Safety:** Collimate to the soft tissue of the wrist. Gonadal shielding should be used on all children and on adults of childbearing age.

- **Position:** Place the patient in a seated position at a table with the wrist placed in the PA position. Instruct the patient to make a loose fist to place the carpal bones closer to the film.

- **Central Ray:** Perpendicular to the film and centered to the midwrist region.

- **Respiration:** Suspended expiration.

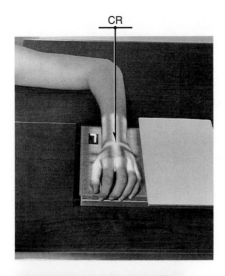

Figure 7–45. PA wrist.

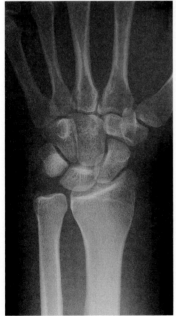

Figure 7–46. PA wrist.

► OBLIQUE WRIST

- **Anatomy:** Distal radius and ulna, lunate, scaphoid, trapezoid, and trapezium.

- **Indication:** This is considered a basic view of the wrist and should be performed with all wrist series.

- **Film:** 8 × 10 in. or 10 × 12 in. crosswise without a grid. The film should be divided into half or thirds to include more than one view.

- **Tube Tilt:** None.

- **FFD:** 40 in.

- **Safety:** Collimate to the soft tissue of the wrist. Gonadal shielding should be used on all children and on adults of childbearing age.

- **Position:** Place the patient in a seated position at a table with the wrist in a PA position. Instruct the patient to move the wrist to a 45° angle to the film, with the ulnar side closest to the film.

- **Central Ray:** Perpendicular to the film and centered to the midwrist region.

- **Respiration:** Suspended expiration.

- **Notes:** A positioning sponge may be used to maintain the wrist at a 45° angle.

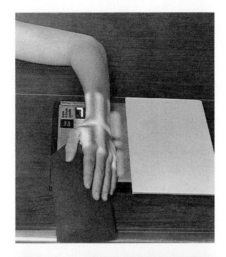

Figure 7–47. Oblique wrist.

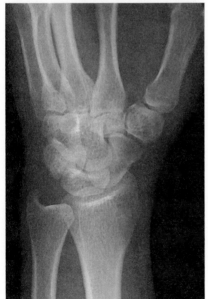

Figure 7–48. Oblique wrist.

► LATERAL WRIST

- **Anatomy:** Trapezium, scaphoid, capitate, lunate, and distal radius and ulna.

- **Indication:** This is considered a basic view of the wrist and should be performed with all wrist series. This view is indicated when a subluxation of the capitate and lunate are suspected.

- **Film:** 8 × 10 in. or 10 × 12 in. crosswise without a grid. The film should be divided in half or thirds to include more than one view.

- **Tube Tilt:** None.

- **FFD:** 40 in.

- **Safety:** Collimate to the soft tissue of the wrist. Gonadal shielding should be used on all children and on adults of childbearing age.

- **Position:** Place the patient in a seated position at a table with the wrist in a true lateral position. Instruct the patient to flex the elbow to 90° with the ulnar side closest to the film.

- **Central Ray:** Perpendicular to the film and centered to the midwrist region.

- **Respiration:** Suspended expiration.

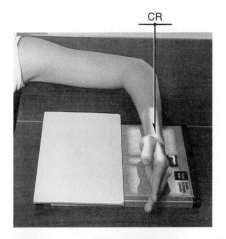

Figure 7–49. Lateral wrist.

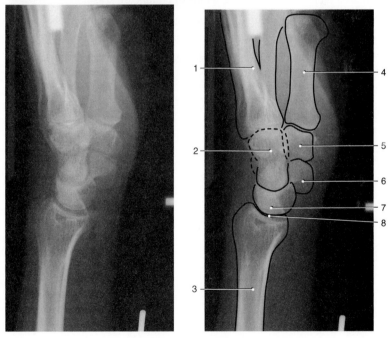

Figure 7–50. Lateral wrist.

► ULNAR FLEXION WRIST (RADIAL DEVIATION)— SCAPHOID VIEW

- **Anatomy:** Distal radius and ulna, scaphoid, lunate, triquetrium, pisiform, trapezium, trapezoid, capitate, and hamate.

- **Indication:** This is an optional view indicated when there is a suspected fracture or nonunion of the scaphoid.

- **Film:** 8 × 10 in. lengthwise without a grid.

- **Tube Tilt:** 10° to 15° along the long axis of the forearm.

- **FFD:** 40 in.

- **Safety:** Collimate to the soft tissue of the wrist. Gonadal shielding should be used on all children and on adults of childbearing age.

- **Position:** Place the patient in a seated position at the table with the wrist in a PA position. Instruct the patient to flex the wrist towards the ulnar side.

- **Central Ray:** 10° to 15° along the long axis of the forearm and centered to the scaphoid.

- **Respiration:** Suspended expiration.

CR

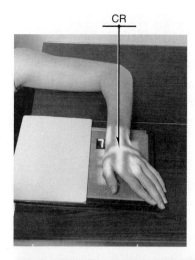

Figure 7–51. Ulnar flexion wrist—scaphoid view.

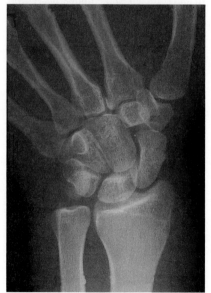

Figure 7–52. Ulnar flexion wrist—scaphoid view.

► RADIAL FLEXION WRIST (ULNAR DEVIATION)

- **Anatomy:** Distal radius and ulna, hamate, pisiform, triquetrum, and lunate.
- **Indication:** This is an optional view taken when there is suspected pathology on the medial side of the carpal bones.
- **Film:** 8 × 10 in. lengthwise without a grid.
- **Tube Tilt:** None.
- **FFD:** 40 in.
- **Safety:** Collimate to the soft tissue of the wrist. Gonadal shielding should be used on all children and on adults of childbearing age.
- **Position:** The patient should be seated at the table with the wrist placed in a PA position. Have the patient flex the wrist towards the radial side.
- **Central Ray:** Perpendicular to the film and directed to the midcarpal region.
- **Respiration:** Suspended expiration.

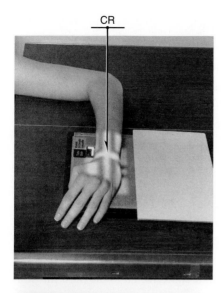

Figure 7–53. Radial flexion wrist.

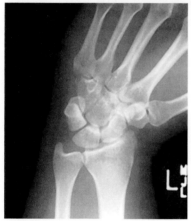

Figure 7–54. Radial flexion wrist.

► PA HAND

- **Anatomy:** Phalanges, metacarpals, and carpals.

- **Indication:** This is considered a basic view of the hand and should be performed with all hand series.

- **Film:** 10 × 12 in. crosswise without a grid. The film should be divided in half to include two views.

- **Tube Tilt:** None.

- **FFD:** 40 in.

- **Safety:** Collimate to the soft tissue of the hand and wrist. Gonadal shielding should be used on all children and on adults of childbearing age.

- **Position:** Place the patient in a seated position at a table with the hand in a PA position on the film (palm down).

- **Central Ray:** Perpendicular to the film and centered to the third metacarpophalangeal joint.

- **Respiration:** Suspended expiration.

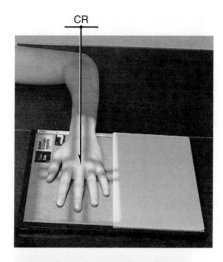

Figure 7–55. PA hand.

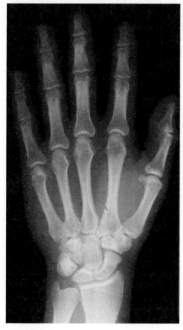

Figure 7–56. PA hand.

► OBLIQUE HAND

- **Anatomy:** Phalanges, metacarpals, and carpals.

- **Indication:** This is considered a basic view and should be performed with all hand series.

- **Film:** 10 × 12 in. crosswise without a grid. The film should be divided in half to include two views.

- **Tube Tilt:** None.

- **FFD:** 40 in.

- **Safety:** Collimate to the soft tissue of the hand and wrist. Gonadal shielding should be used on all children and on adults of childbearing age.

- **Position:** Place the patient in a seated position at a table with the hand in a PA position on the film (palm down). Instruct the patient to hold the hand at a 45° angle, with the ulnar side closest to the film. A step block sponge may be used to separate the digits in the oblique position.

- **Central Ray:** Perpendicular to the film and centered to the third metacarpophalangeal joint.

- **Respiration:** Suspended expiration.

- **Notes:** The patient may make an "okay" sign with the thumb and second digit to support the hand if a step block positioning sponge is not used.

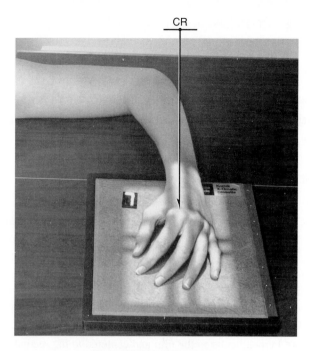

Figure 7–57. Oblique hand.

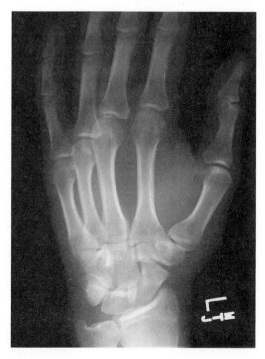

Figure 7–58. Oblique hand.

► LATERAL HAND

- **Anatomy:** Phalanges, metacarpal/phalangeal joints, and carpals.

- **Indication:** This is considered a basic view of the hand and should be performed with all hand series.

- **Film:** 8 × 10 in. lengthwise without a grid.

- **Tube Tilt:** None.

- **FFD:** 40 in.

- **Safety:** Collimate to the soft tissue of the hand and wrist. Gonadal shielding should be used on all children and on adults of childbearing age.

- **Position:** Place the patient in a seated position at a table with the hand in a true lateral position. The ulnar side of the hand should be placed closest to the film. Instruct the patient to fan the fingers so that they are not superimposed. This may be achieved by using a step block sponge to support the hand.

- **Central Ray:** Perpendicular to the film and centered to the second metacarpophalangeal joint.

- **Respiration:** Suspended expiration.

- **Notes:** The patient may make an "okay" sign with the thumb and second digit; however, make sure the hand is kept in a true lateral position.

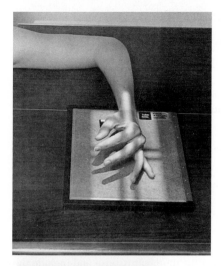

Figure 7–59. Lateral hand.

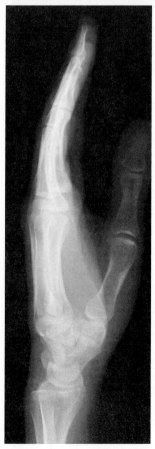

Figure 7–60. Lateral hand.

► AP THUMB

- **Anatomy:** Distal and proximal phalanx, first metacarpal, interphalangeal joint, metacarpal/phalangeal joint, first carpal/metacarpal joint, trapezium, and sesamoid bones.

- **Indication:** This is considered a basic view of the thumb and should be performed with all thumb series.

- **Film:** 8 × 10 in. crosswise without a grid. The film should be divided into thirds to include three views.

- **Tube Tilt:** None.

- **FFD:** 40 in.

- **Safety:** Collimate to the soft tissue of the thumb crosswise and include the trapezium of the wrist lengthwise. Gonadal shielding should be used on all children and on adults of childbearing age.

- **Position:** Place the patient in a seated position at a table with the hand internally rotated so that the thumbnail is placed on the film. Make sure the fingers are extended back out of the way.

- **Central Ray:** Perpendicular to the film and centered to the first metacarpophalangeal joint.

- **Respiration:** Suspended expiration.

- **Notes:** A PA view of the thumb may be performed if the patient is unable to place the thumb in an AP position. This is achieved by placing the hand in a lateral position and supporting the thumb in a PA position with a positioning sponge. This does increase object film distance, which causes magnification.

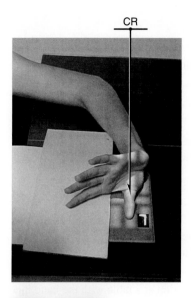

Figure 7–61. AP thumb.

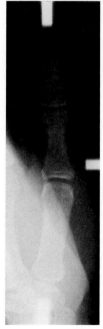

Figure 7–62. AP thumb.

▶ LATERAL THUMB

- **Anatomy:** Distal phalanx, proximal phalanx, first metacarpal, trapezium, sesamoid bones, interphalangeal joint, metacarpal/phalangeal joint, and first carpal/metacarpal joint.

- **Indication:** This is considered a basic view of the thumb and should be performed with all thumb series.

- **Film:** 8 × 10 in. crosswise without a grid. The film should be divided into thirds to include three views.

- **Tube Tilt:** None.

- **FFD:** 40 in.

- **Safety:** Collimate to the soft tissue of the thumb crosswise and include the trapezium lengthwise. Gonadal shielding should be used on all children and on adults of childbearing age.

- **Position:** Place the patient in a seated position at a table with the hand in a PA position. Instruct the patient to internally rotate the hand until the thumb is in a true lateral position.

- **Central Ray:** Perpendicular to the film and centered to the first metacarpophalangeal joint.

- **Respiration:** Suspended expiration.

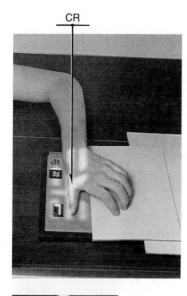

Figure 7–63. Lateral thumb.

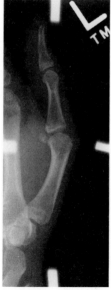

Figure 7–64. Lateral thumb.

▶ OBLIQUE THUMB

- **Anatomy:** Distal phalanx, proximal phalanx, first metacarpal, trapezium, first carpal/metacarpal joint, first metacarpal/phalangeal joint, interphalangeal joint, and sesamoid bones.

- **Indication:** This is considered a basic view of the thumb and should be performed with all thumb series.

- **Film:** 8 × 10 in. crosswise without a grid. The film should be divided into thirds to include three views.

- **Tube Tilt:** None.

- **FFD:** 40 in.

- **Safety:** Collimate to the soft tissue of the thumb crosswise and include the trapezium lengthwise. Gonadal shielding should be used on all children and on adults of childbearing age.

- **Position:** Place the patient in a seated position at a table with the hand in a PA position (palm down). This places the thumb in a 45° angle with the film.

- **Central Ray:** Perpendicular to the film and centered to the first metacarpophalangeal joint.

- **Respiration:** Suspended expiration.

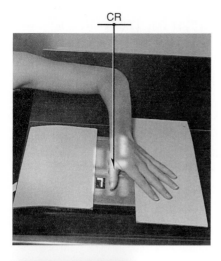

Figure 7–65. Oblique thumb.

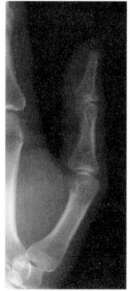

Figure 7–66. Oblique thumb.

▶ PA SECOND THROUGH FIFTH DIGITS

- **Anatomy:** Distal, middle and proximal phalanx, distal interphalangeal joints, proximal interphalangeal joints, metacarpophalangeal joints, and metacarpals.

- **Indication:** This is considered a basic view of the digits and should be performed with all finger series.

- **Film:** 8 × 10 in. crosswise without a grid. The film should be divided into thirds for three views.

- **Tube Tilt:** None.

- **FFD:** 40 in.

- **Safety:** Collimate to the soft tissue of the finger of interest crosswise and include the distal metacarpal lengthwise.

- **Position:** Place the patient in a seated position at a table with the hand in a PA position (palm down).

- **Central Ray:** Perpendicular to the film and centered to the proximal interphalangeal joint of the digit being x-rayed.

- **Respiration:** Suspended expiration.

CR

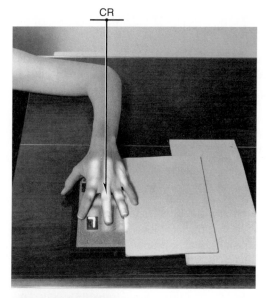

Figure 7–67. PA third digit.

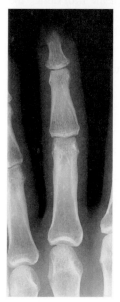

Figure 7–68. PA third digit.

▶ LATERAL SECOND THROUGH FIFTH DIGITS

- **Anatomy:** Distal, middle and proximal phalanx, distal interphalangeal joint, proximal interphalangeal joint, and metacarpal/phalangeal joints.

- **Indication:** This is considered a basic view and should be performed with all finger series.

- **Film:** 8 × 10 in. crosswise without a grid. The film should be divided into thirds to include three views.

- **Tube Tilt:** None.

- **FFD:** 40 in.

- **Safety:** Collimate to the soft tissue of the finger of interest crosswise and include the distal metacarpal lengthwise. Gonadal shielding should be used on all children and on adults of childbearing age.

- **Position:** Place the patient in a seated position at a table with the hand in a true lateral position. For the second digit, the radial side of the finger should be closest to the film. For the third through the fifth digits, the ulnar side of the digits should be closest to the film. The long axis of the digit should be parallel to the film and all other digits moved to avoid superimposition.

- **Central Ray:** Perpendicular to the film and centered to the proximal interphalangeal joint.

- **Respiration:** Suspended expiration.

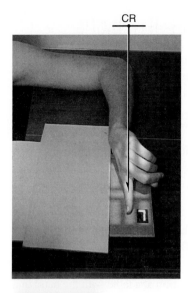

Figure 7–69. Lateral second digit.

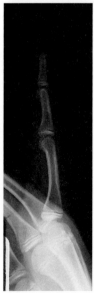

Figure 7–70. Lateral second digit.

► OBLIQUE SECOND THROUGH FIFTH DIGITS

- **Anatomy:** Distal, middle and proximal phalanx, distal interphalangeal joint, proximal interphalangeal joint, metacarpophalangeal joint, and metacarpals.

- **Indication:** This is considered a basic view of the digits and should be performed with all finger series.

- **Film:** 8 × 10 in. crosswise without a grid. The film should be divided into thirds to include three views.

- **Tube Tilt:** None.

- **FFD:** 40 in.

- **Safety:** Collimate to the soft tissue of the finger of interest and the distal metacarpal lengthwise. Gonadal shielding should be used on all children and on adults of childbearing age.

- **Position:** Place the patient in a seated position at a table with the hand in a PA position (palm down). The digits should be at a 45° angle with the film. The second digit should be positioned medially, with the radial side closest to the film. The third through the fifth digits should be positioned laterally, with the ulnar side closest to the film.

- **Central Ray:** Perpendicular to the film and centered to the proximal interphalangeal joint.

- **Respiration:** Suspended expiration.

- **Notes:** Make sure that the other digits are moved out of the way to avoid superimposition.

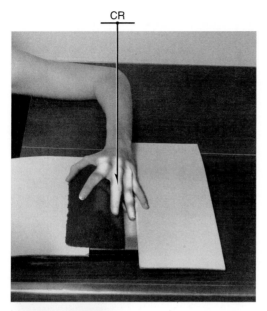

Figure 7–71. Oblique third digit.

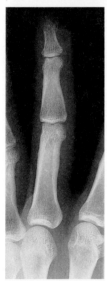

Figure 7–72. Oblique third digit.

LOWER EXTREMITY RADIOGRAPHY

8

► AP PELVIS

- **Anatomy:** Iliac crest, ilium, sacroiliac joints, sacrum, symphysis pubis, obturator foramen, and femoral heads.

- **Indication:** This is considered a basic view of the pelvis and should be performed with all pelvic series.

- **Film:** 14 × 17 in. crosswise with a grid.

- **Tube Tilt:** None.

- **FFD:** 40 in.

- **Safety:** Collimate to an area slightly less than the size of film being used. Gonadal shielding should be used when possible without obscuring anatomy (male patients).

- **Position:** Place the patient in an upright position with the back against the film. Internally rotate the feet 15° in order to place the femoral head in a true AP position. This view may be done with the patient supine.

- **Central Ray:** Perpendicular to the film and centered to midpelvis, which is approximately 2 in. superior to the symphysis pubis.

- **Respiration:** Suspended expiration.

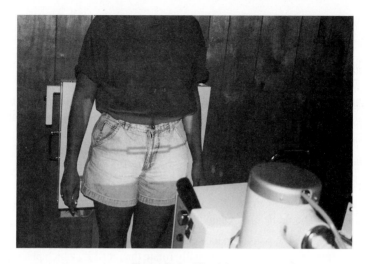

Figure 8–1. AP pelvis.

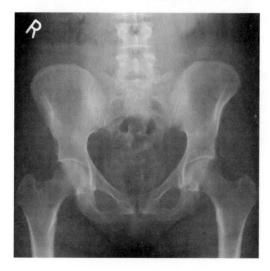

Figure 8–2. AP pelvis.

► AP HIP

- **Anatomy:** Femoral head, femoral neck, greater trochanter, intertrocanteric crest, lesser trochanter, and acetabulum.

- **Indication:** This is considered a basic view and should be performed with all hip series. If a fracture is suspected, then a CT scan may be indicated.

- **Film:** 8 × 10 in. lengthwise with a grid.

- **Tube Tilt:** None.

- **FFD:** 40 in.

- **Safety:** Collimate to an area slightly less than the film being used. Gonadal shielding should be used when possible without obscuring anatomy.

- **Position:** Place the patient in an upright position with the back against the film. Instruct the patient to internally rotate the foot 15°, which places the hip in an AP position. This view may be done with the patient supine.

- **Central Ray:** Perpendicular to the film and centered to the femoral neck.

- **Respiration:** Suspended expiration.

- **Notes:**
  1. The femoral neck may be located by drawing an imaginary line from the ASIS to the symphysis pubis, dividing it in half, and dropping down approximately 2.5 in. from the midpoint of this imaginary line.
  2. A true AP projection of the hip (with 15° internal rotation of the foot) will allow the practitioner to visualize the greater trochanter.

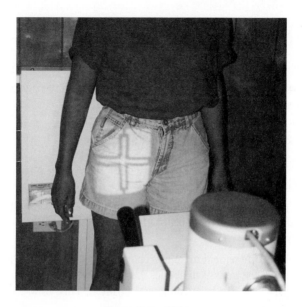

Figure 8–3. AP hip.

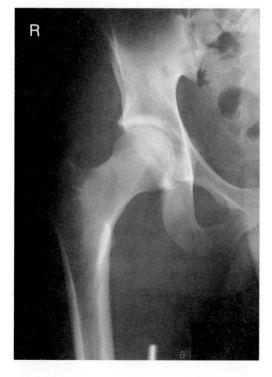

Figure 8–4. AP hip.

▶ LATERAL HIP—FROG-LEG VIEW

- **Anatomy:** Acetabulum, femoral head, femoral neck, and lesser trochanter.
- **Indication:** This is considered a basic view and should be performed with all hip series. If the patient is unable to sustain the position needed to perform this view, then a CT scan may be indicated.
- **Film:** 8 × 10 in. lengthwise with a grid.
- **Tube Tilt:** None.
- **FFD:** 40 in.
- **Safety:** Collimate to an area slightly less than the size of film being used. Gonadal shielding should be used when possible without obscuring anatomy.
- **Position:** Place the patient in an upright position with the back against the film. Instruct the patient to abduct the femur and flex the hip and knee, which places the hip in a true lateral position. This view may be done with the patient supine.
- **Central Ray:** Perpendicular to the film and centered to the femoral neck.
- **Respiration:** Suspended expiration.
- **Notes:**
  1. This view is best done with the patient in a supine position so the patient does not lose his or her balance.
  2. This view allows the practitioner to visualize the lesser trochanter.

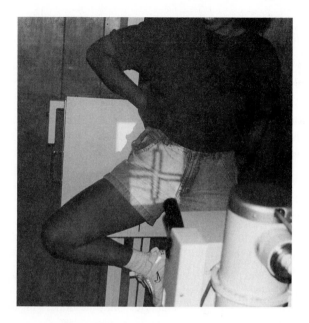

Figure 8–5. Lateral hip—frog-leg view.

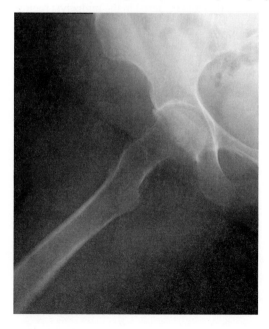

Figure 8–6. Lateral hip—frog-leg view.

▶ BILATERAL AP HIPS

- **Anatomy:** Pelvis, sacrum, coccyx, symphysis pubis, ischial tuberosities, femoral heads, femoral necks, greater trochanters, and intertrochanteric crest.

- **Indication:** This view is indicated when comparison of the normal and affected hip is needed, or in the evaluation of certain pathologies that affect both joints, such as rheumatoid arthritis.

- **Film:** 14 × 17 in. crosswise with a grid.

- **Tube Tilt:** None.

- **FFD:** 40 in.

- **Safety:** Collimate to an area slightly less than the film being used. Gonadal shielding should be used when possible without obscuring anatomy.

- **Position:** Place the patient in an upright position with the back against the film. Instruct the patient to internally rotate the feet 15°, which places the hips in an true AP position. This view may be done with the patient supine.

- **Central Ray:** Perpendicular to the film and centered to the midpelvis region.

- **Respiration:** Suspended expiration.

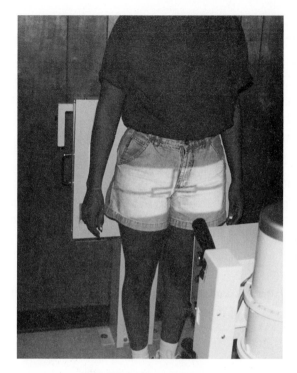

Figure 8–7. Bilateral AP hips.

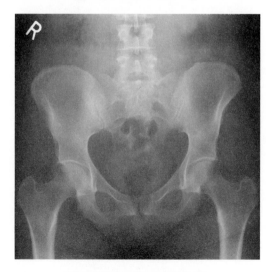

Figure 8–8. Bilateral AP hips.

▶ BILATERAL HIPS—FROG-LEG VIEW

- **Anatomy:** Pelvis, sacrum, coccyx, ischial tuberosities, obturator foramen, femoral heads, femoral necks, and lesser trochanters.

- **Indication:** This view is indicated when comparison views of the hips are needed or pathology that affects both joints is suspected.

- **Film:** 14 × 17 in. crosswise with a grid.

- **Tube Tilt:** None.

- **FFD:** 40 in.

- **Safety:** Collimate to an area slightly less than the film being used. Gonadal shielding should be used when possible without obscuring anatomy.

- **Position:** Place the patient in a supine position with the back against the film. Instruct the patient to flex the hips and knees bilaterally and abduct both femurs.

- **Central Ray:** Perpendicular to the film and centered to the midpelvis region.

- **Respiration:** Suspended expiration.

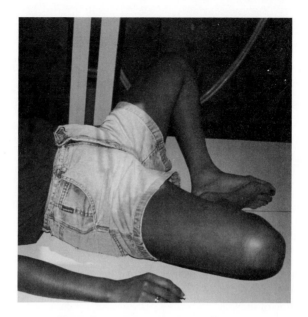

Figure 8–9. Bilateral hips—frog-leg view.

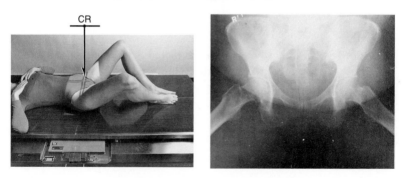

Figure 8–10. Bilateral hips—frog-leg view.

▶ AP FEMUR

- **Anatomy:** Shaft of the femur, hip joint, knee joint, and femoral epicondyles.

- **Indication:** This is considered a basic view of the femur and should be performed with all femoral series.

- **Film:** 14 × 17 in. lengthwise with a grid.

- **Tube Tilt:** None.

- **FFD:** 40 in.

- **Safety:** Collimate to the soft tissue of the thigh crosswise and include the hip and knee joint lengthwise. Gonadal shielding should be used with all patients as long as the anatomy is not obscured.

- **Position:** Place the patient in an upright position with the back against the film. The intercondylar line should be parallel to the film when the femur is placed in a true AP position. This may require approximately 5° internal rotation of the leg.

- **Central Ray:** Perpendicular to the film and centered to the midshaft of the femur.

- **Respiration:** Suspended expiration.

- **Notes:** Make sure that both joints are included in x-rays of the femur, because the femur helps form both the hip and knee joints. This usually requires that an AP and lateral hip series be taken separately.

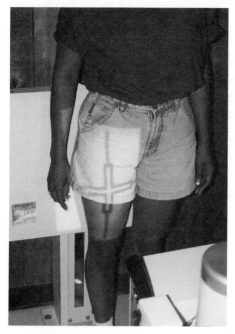

Figure 8–11. AP femur.

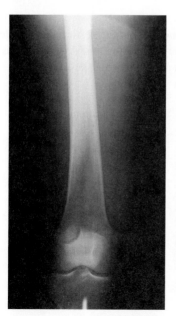

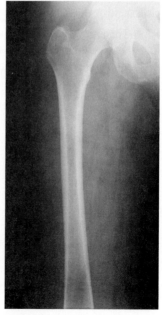

Figure 8–12. AP femur.

► LATERAL FEMUR

- **Anatomy:** Shaft of the femur, knee joint, and hip joint.

- **Indication:** This is considered a basic view of the femur and should be performed with all femoral series.

- **Film:** 14 × 17 in. lengthwise with a grid.

- **Tube Tilt:** None.

- **FFD:** 40 in.

- **Safety:** Collimate to an area slightly less than the size of film being used. Gonadal shielding should be used on all patients without the anatomy being obscured.

- **Position:** Place the patient in an upright position with the affected side against the film in a lateral position. Instruct the patient to move the unaffected leg out of the field of view. The intercondylar line should be placed perpendicular to the film. This view may be done with the patient recumbent.

- **Central Ray:** Perpendicular to the film and centered to the midshaft of the femur.

- **Respiration:** Suspended expiration.

- **Notes:** The lateral view of the femur should be performed in order to include the knee joint. A frog-leg hip view should be done since it is impossible to include the hip joint on a lateral femur view.

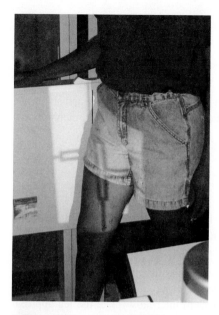

Figure 8–13. Lateral femur.

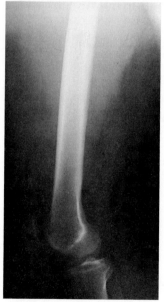

Figure 8–14. Lateral femur.

► AP/PA KNEE

- **Anatomy:** Patella, femoral condyles, tibial plateau, head of the fibula, tibia, and femorotibial joint space.

- **Indication:** This view is considered a basic view of the knee and should be performed with all knee series. If an abnormality is present, then optional views may be indicated.

- **Film:** 8 × 10 in. or 10 ×12 in. lengthwise with or without a grid.

- **Tube Tilt:** 5° cephalad.

- **FFD:** 40 in.

- **Safety:** Collimate to soft tissue of the knee crosswise and slightly less than the length of film being used. Gonadal shielding should be used on all children and on adults of childbearing age.

- **Position:** Place the patient in an upright position with the back against the film. The intercondylar line of the femur should be placed parallel to the film, which may require the patient to internally rotate the leg approximately 5° to place the knee in a true AP position. This view may be done with the patient supine.

- **Central Ray:** 5° cephalad and centered one-half inch inferior to the patellar apex.

- **Respiration:** Suspended expiration.

- **Notes:** This view may be done in a PA position with the patient facing the film. In a PA position, the tibia and fibula are at a slight inclination, which places the central ray perpendicular to the tibial plateau without a tube tilt.

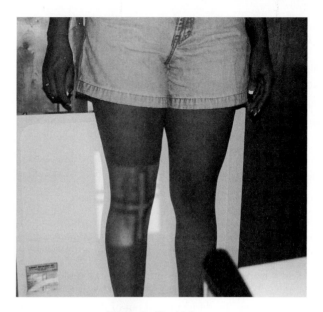

Figure 8–15. AP knee.

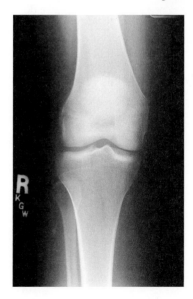

Figure 8–16. AP knee.

► LATERAL KNEE

- **Anatomy:** Patella, patellofemoral joint, distal femur, proximal tibia, proximal fibula, and femoral epicondyles superimposed.

- **Indication:** This is considered a basic view of the knee and should be performed with all knee series. If an abnormality is present, then optional views may be indicated.

- **Film:** 8 × 10 in. or 10 ×12 in. lengthwise with or without a grid.

- **Tube Tilt:** 5° cephalad.

- **FFD:** 40 in.

- **Safety:** Collimate to the soft tissue of the knee crosswise and slightly less than the length of film being used. Gonadal shielding should be used on all children and on adults of childbearing age.

- **Position:** Place the patient in an upright position. Instruct the patient to flex the knee 45° with the affected knee against the film in a lateral position. The unaffected knee should be moved out of the way. This view may be done with the patient recumbent.

- **Central Ray:** 5° cephalad and centered one-half inch distal to the medial epicondyle.

- **Respiration:** Suspended expiration.

- **Notes:** Notice that the medial epicondyle appears larger than the lateral epicondyle due to magnification.

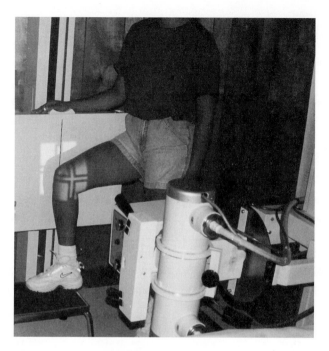

Figure 8–17. Lateral knee.

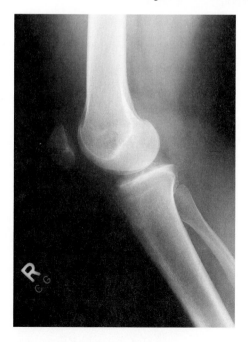

Figure 8–18. Lateral knee.

▶ MEDIAL OBLIQUE KNEE

- **Anatomy:** Distal femur, patella, condyles of the femur, fibular head and neck, tibia, and proximal tibiofibular joint.

- **Indication:** This view is indicated when a fracture of the proximal fibular head or neck region is suspected. This view places the fibular head and neck in a position without superimposition of the tibia.

- **Film:** 8 × 10 in. or 10 ×12 in. lengthwise with or without a grid.

- **Tube Tilt:** None.

- **FFD:** 40 in.

- **Safety:** Collimate to the soft tissue of the knee crosswise and slightly less than the length of film being used. Gonadal shielding should be used on all children and on adults of childbearing age.

- **Position:** Place the patient in an upright position with the back against the film. Instruct the patient to internally rotate the leg 45°. This view may be done with the patient recumbent.

- **Central Ray:** Perpendicular to the film and centered one-half inch below the patellar apex.

- **Respiration:** Suspended expiration.

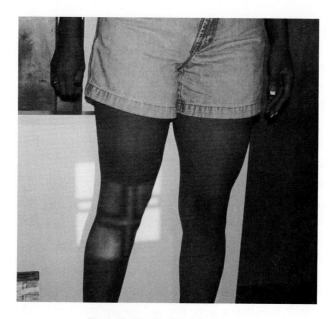

Figure 8–19. Medial oblique knee.

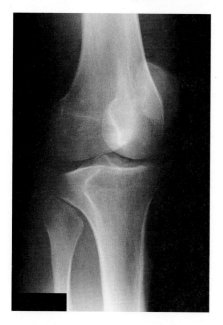

Figure 8–20. Medial oblique knee.

▶ LATERAL (EXTERNAL) OBLIQUE KNEE

- **Anatomy:** Patella, distal femur, femoral condyles, tibial condyles, tibial plateau, and proximal fibula and tibia.

- **Indication:** This view is an optional view and is obtained to visualize the lateral tibiofemoral joint space.

- **Film:** 8 × 10 in. or 10 × 12 in. lengthwise with or without a grid.

- **Tube Tilt:** None.

- **FFD:** 40 in.

- **Safety:** Collimate to the soft tissue of the knee crosswise and slightly less than the length of film being used. Gonadal shielding should be used on all children and on adults of childbearing age.

- **Position:** Place the patient in an upright position with the back against the film. Instruct the patient to externally rotate the leg 45°. This view may be done with the patient recumbent.

- **Central Ray:** Perpendicular to the film and centered one-half inch below the patellar apex.

- **Respiration:** Suspended expiration.

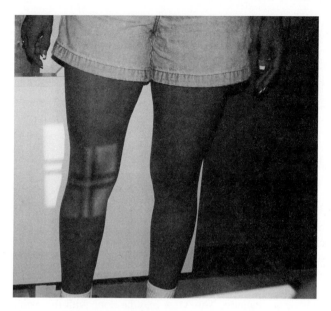

Figure 8–21. Lateral (external) oblique knee.

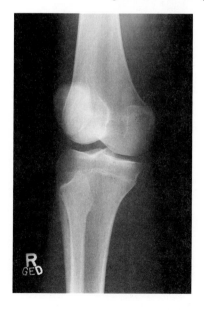

Figure 8–22. Lateral (external) oblique knee.

▶ PA AXIAL KNEE—TUNNEL VIEW

- **Anatomy:** Patella, intercondylar fossa, femoral condyles, tibial condyles, and intercondylar fossa.

- **Indication:** This view is considered an optional view and is taken when pathology (such as joint mice) is suspected in the intercondylar fossas.

- **Film:** 8 × 10 in. lengthwise without a grid.

- **Tube Tilt:** 45° cephalad.

- **FFD:** 40 in.

- **Safety:** Collimate to the soft tissue of the knee crosswise and slightly less than the length of film being used. Gonadal shielding should be used on all children and on adults of childbearing age.

- **Position:** Place the patient in an upright position with the knee flexed 45° and resting on a stool. The film is placed underneath the patient's knee. Make sure that the patient has a stationary object to hold on to in order to keep his or her balance. This view may be done with the patient prone and the lower leg elevated 45°.

- **Central Ray:** With the patient erect: 45° cephalad and centered to the midpoint of the popliteal fossa. With the patient prone: 45° caudad and centered to the midpoint of the popliteal fossa.

- **Respiration:** Suspended expiration.

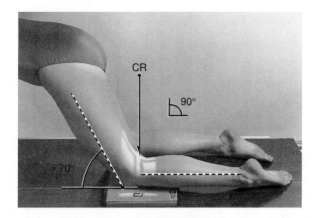

Figure 8–23. PA axial knee—tunnel view.

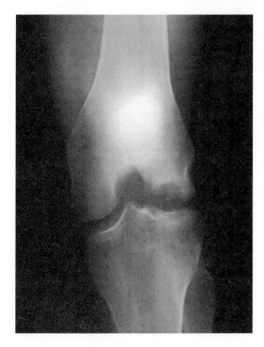

Figure 8–24. PA axial knee —tunnel view.

▶ TANGENTIAL KNEE—SUNRISE VIEW

- **Anatomy:** Patella, patellofemoral joint space, and femoral condyles.

- **Indication:** This is an optional view that is indicated when pathology is suspected of the patella.

- **Film:** 8 × 10 in. lengthwise without a grid.

- **Tube Tilt:** Perpendicular to the patella depending on how much flexion the patient can achieve with the knee.

- **FFD:** 40 in.

- **Safety:** Collimate to an area to include the soft tissue of the patella, approximately 4 × 4 in. Gonadal shielding should be used on all children and on adults of childbearing age.

- **Position:** Place the patient in a seated position with the knee flexed as much as tolerable. Instruct the patient to hold the film against the femur. A tube tilt is then used in order to place the central ray perpendicular to the patella or parallel to the patellofemoral joint space.

- **Central Ray:** Perpendicular to the patella (which requires a tube tilt) and centered to the patella.

- **Respiration:** Suspended expiration.

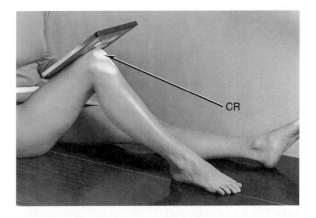

Figure 8–25. Tangential knee—sunrise view.

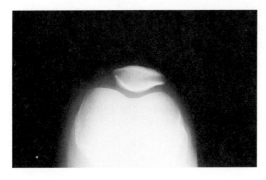

Figure 8–26. Tangential knee —sunrise view.

▶ BILATERAL WEIGHT BEARING KNEES

- **Anatomy:** Bilateral knees to include the proximal tibia and fibula, distal femur, patella, tibiofemoral joint space, and tibial plateau.

- **Indication:** This view is recommended when arthritides are suspected of the knees.

- **Film:** 14 × 17 in. crosswise with or without a grid.

- **Tube Tilt:** 5° cephalad.

- **FFD:** 40 in.

- **Safety:** Collimate to an area to include the soft tissue of both knees. Gonadal shielding should be used on all children and on adults of child-bearing age.

- **Position:** Place the patient in an upright position with the back against the film. The patient may be placed on a stepstool in order to raise the knees to be centered on the film.

- **Central Ray:** 5° cephalad and centered to the film.

- **Respiration:** Suspended expiration.

- **Notes:** Make sure that the patient evenly distributes his or her weight on both feet.

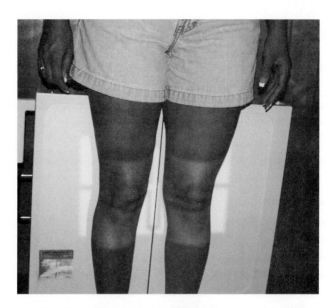

Figure 8–27. Bilateral weight bearing knees.

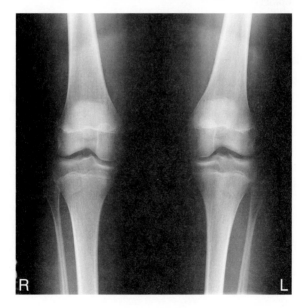

Figure 8–28. Bilateral weight bearing knees.

▶ AP LOWER LEG

- **Anatomy:** Knee joint, tibia, fibula, medial and lateral malleolus, and ankle joint.

- **Indication:** This is considered a basic view of the lower leg and should be performed with all lower leg series.

- **Film:** 14 × 17 in. lengthwise without a grid. The film should be divided in half to include two views.

- **Tube Tilt:** None.

- **FFD:** 40 in.

- **Safety:** Collimate to the soft tissue of the lower leg crosswise and slightly less than the length of film being used. Gonadal shielding should be used on all children and on adults of childbearing age.

- **Position:** Place the patient in an upright position with the back against the film. The intermalleolar line should be parallel to the film, which may require slight rotation of the lower leg. This view may be done with the patient supine.

- **Central Ray:** Perpendicular to the film and centered to the midshaft of the tibia.

- **Respiration:** Suspended expiration.

- **Notes:** Make sure that the knee joint and the ankle joint are both included on the film. If both joints cannot be achieved on one film, then separate AP views should be done of each joint.

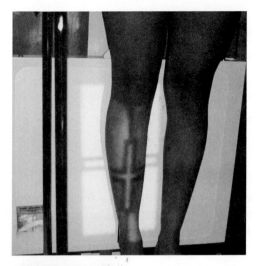

Figure 8–29. AP lower leg.

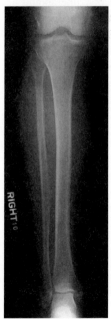

Figure 8–30. AP lower leg.

▶ LATERAL LOWER LEG

- **Anatomy:** Knee joint, tibia, fibula, ankle joint, and patella.

- **Indication:** This is considered a basic view of the lower leg and should be performed with all lower leg series.

- **Film:** 14 × 17 in. lengthwise without a grid. The film should be divided in half to include two views.

- **Tube Tilt:** None.

- **FFD:** 40 in.

- **Safety:** Collimate to the soft tissue of the lower leg crosswise and slightly less than the length of film being used. Gonadal shielding should be used on all children and on adults of childbearing age.

- **Position:** Place the patient in an upright position with the affected leg against the film in a lateral position. The intermalleolar line should be placed perpendicular to the film. Make sure that the unaffected leg is moved out of the way to avoid superimposition. Instruct the patient to flex the knee approximately 45°. This view may be done with the patient recumbent.

- **Central Ray:** Perpendicular to the film and centered to the midshaft of the tibia.

- **Respiration:** Suspended expiration.

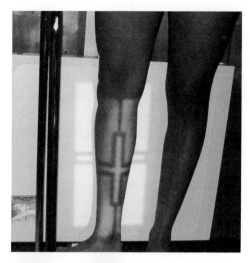

Figure 8–31. Lateral lower leg.

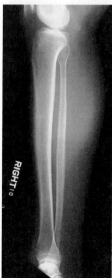

Figure 8–32. Lateral lower leg.

► AP ANKLE

- **Anatomy:** Medial and lateral malleolus, distal tibiofibular joint, and talus.
- **Indication:** This is considered a basic view of the ankle and should be performed with all ankle series. If an abnormality is present, optional views may be indicated.
- **Film:** 10 × 12 in. crosswise without a grid. The film should be divided in half for two views.
- **Tube Tilt:** None.
- **FFD:** 40 in.
- **Safety:** Collimate to the soft tissue of the ankle crosswise and slightly less than the length of the film being used. Gonadal shielding should be used on all children and on adults of childbearing age.
- **Position:** Place the patient in a seated position with the ankle joint placed in a true AP position. Instruct the patient to dorsiflex the foot. The intermalleolar line should be parallel to the film, which may require slight internal rotation of the foot.
- **Central Ray:** Perpendicular to the film and centered to the midpoint of the ankle.
- **Respiration:** Suspended expiration.

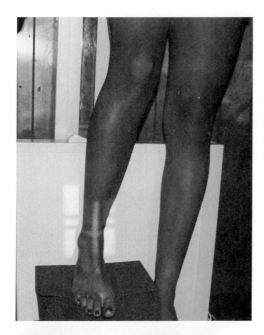

Figure 8–33. AP ankle.

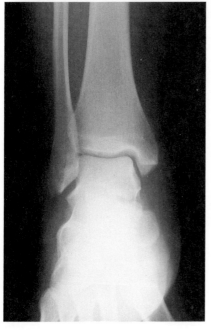

Figure 8–34. AP ankle.

► LATERAL ANKLE

- **Anatomy:** Distal tibia and fibula, talus, tarsal sinus, calcaneus, and talonavicular joint space.

- **Indication:** This is considered a basic view of the ankle and should be performed with all ankle series. If an abnormality is present, optional views may be indicated.

- **Film:** 10 × 12 in. crosswise without a grid. The film should be divided in half for two views.

- **Tube Tilt:** None.

- **FFD:** 40 in.

- **Safety:** Collimate to the soft tissue of the ankle crosswise and slightly less than the length of film being used. Gonadal shielding should be used on all children and on adults of childbearing age.

- **Position:** Place the patient in a seated position with the ankle internally rotated 45°. Instruct the patient to dorsiflex the foot as much as possible.

- **Central Ray:** Perpendicular to the film and centered to the midankle joint.

- **Respiration:** Suspended expiration.

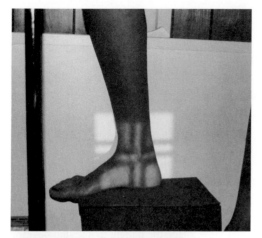

Figure 8–35. Lateral ankle.

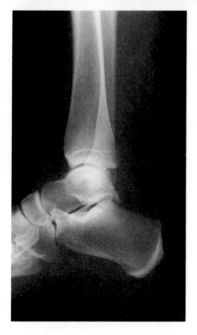

Figure 8–36. Lateral ankle.

▶ MEDIAL AND LATERAL OBLIQUE ANKLE

- **Anatomy:** Distal tibia and fibula, medial and lateral malleolus.

- **Indication:** This view is indicated when the practitioner is attempting to rule out fracture of the talocalcaneal region.

- **Film:** 10 × 12 in. crosswise without a grid.

- **Tube Tilt:** None.

- **FFD:** 40 in.

- **Safety:** Collimate to the soft tissue of the ankle crosswise and slightly less than the length of the film being used. Gonadal shielding should be used on all children and on adults of childbearing age.

- **Position:** For the lateral oblique view, place the patient in a seated position with the ankle rotated 45° externally. For a medial oblique view, rotate the ankle 45° medially. Instruct the patient to dorsiflex the foot as much as possible.

- **Central Ray:** Perpendicular to the film and centered to the midankle joint.

- **Respiration:** Suspended expiration.

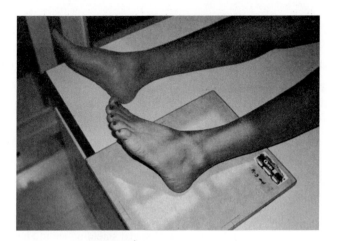

Figure 8–37. Medial oblique ankle.

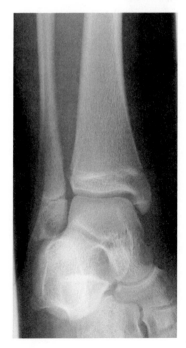

Figure 8–38. Medial oblique ankle.

▶ AP ANKLE—STRESS VIEWS

- **Anatomy:** Distal tibia and fibula, lateral and medial malleolus, and talus.

- **Indication:** This view is indicated to evaluate joint separation and/or ligamentous instability. Inversion of the foot evaluates the lateral ligaments. Eversion of the foot evaluates the medial ligaments.

- **Film:** 10 × 12 in. crosswise without a grid. The film should be divided in half for two views.

- **Tube Tilt:** None.

- **FFD:** 40 in.

- **Safety:** Collimate to the soft tissue of the ankle crosswise and slightly less than the length of film being used. Gonadal shielding should be used on all children and on adults of childbearing age.

- **Position:** Place the patient in a seated position with the ankle placed in a true AP position. The intermalleolar line should be placed parallel to the film. Then place the foot in either an inversion or eversion position, which will place stress on the ankle joint.

- **Central Ray:** Perpendicular to the film and centered to the midankle joint.

- **Respiration:** Suspended expiration.

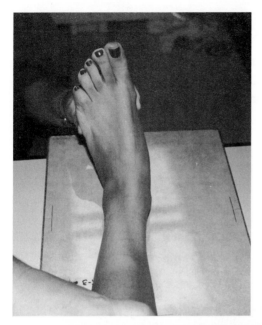

Figure 8–39. AP ankle with eversion stress.

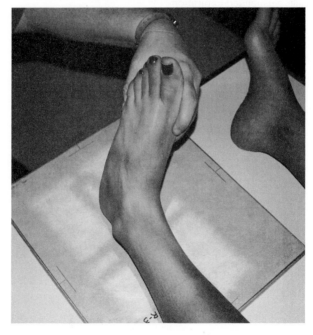

Figure 8–40. AP ankle with inversion stress.

▶ PLANTODORSAL AXIAL CALCANEUS

- **Anatomy:** Calcaneus, sustentaculum tali, and trochlear process.

- **Indication:** This is considered a basic view of the calcaneus and should be done with all calcaneal series.

- **Film:** 8 × 10 in. lengthwise without a grid.

- **Tube Tilt:** 40° cephalad.

- **FFD:** 40 in.

- **Safety:** Collimate to the soft tissue of the calcaneous crosswise and slightly less than the length of film being used. Gonadal shielding should be used on all children and on adults of childbearing age.

- **Position:** Place the patient in a seated position with the foot dorsiflexed as much as possible. Gauze or tape may be used around the foot in order to achieve as much dorsiflexion as possible. Make sure the heel of the foot is placed in the center of the film.

- **Central Ray:** 40° cephalad and centered to the base of the third metatarsal.

- **Respiration:** Suspended expiration.

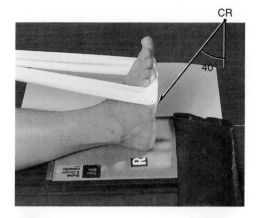

Figure 8–41. Plantodorsal
axial calcaneous.

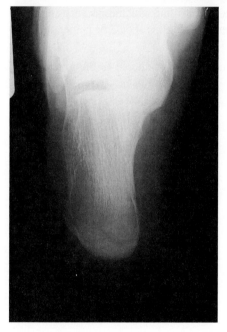

Figure 8–42. Plantodorsal
axial calcaneous.

► LATERAL CALCANEUS

- **Anatomy:** Calcaneus, tibiotalar joint, tarsal sinus, talus, and talonavicular joint.

- **Indication:** This view is considered a basic view and should be performed with all calcaneal series.

- **Film:** 8 × 10 in. lengthwise without a grid.

- **Tube Tilt:** None.

- **FFD:** 40 in.

- **Safety:** Collimate to the soft tissue of the calcaneous. Gonadal shielding should be used on all children and on adults of childbearing age.

- **Position:** Place the patient in a seated position with the calcaneus placed in a true lateral position. The intermalleolar line should be perpendicular to the film.

- **Central Ray:** Perpendicular to the film and centered to the midcalcaneal region.

- **Respiration:** Suspended expiration.

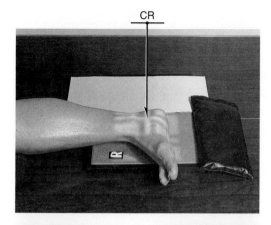

Figure 8–43. Lateral calcaneous.

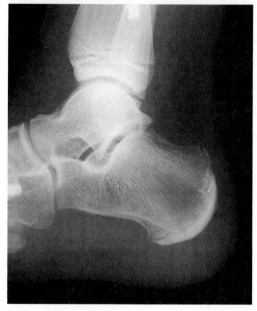

Figure 8–44. Lateral calcaneous.

▶ AP FOOT

- **Anatomy:** Distal, middle and proximal phalanges, interphalangeal joints, sesamoid bones, metatarsals, cuneiforms, cuboid, and navicular.

- **Indication:** This is considered a basic view of the foot and should be performed with all foot series.

- **Film:** 10 × 12 in. crosswise without a grid. The film should be divided in half for two views.

- **Tube Tilt:** 10° towards the heel of the foot.

- **FFD:** 40 in.

- **Safety:** Collimate to the soft tissue of the foot including toes. Gonadal shielding should be used on all children and on adults of childbearing age.

- **Position:** Place the patient in a seated or standing position. Instruct the patient to place the foot on the film as if standing on the sole of the foot.

- **Central Ray:** 10° towards the heel and centered to the base of the third metatarsal.

- **Respiration:** Suspended expiration.

- **Notes:** The central ray requires a tube tilt in order to place it perpendicular to the metatarsals.

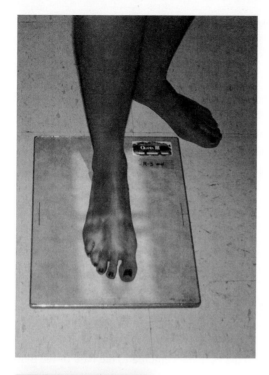

Figure 8–45. AP foot.

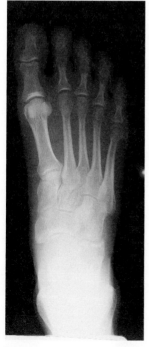

Figure 8–46. AP foot.

► LATERAL FOOT

- **Anatomy:** Calcaneus, talus, navicular, cuboid, first cuneiform, and base of the fifth metarsal.

- **Indication:** This is considered a basic view of the foot and should be performed with all foot series.

- **Film:** 10 × 12 in. crosswise without a grid. The film should be divided in half for two views.

- **Tube Tilt:** None.

- **FFD:** 40 in.

- **Safety:** Collimate to the soft tissue of the foot including toes. Gonadal shielding should be used on all children and on adults of childbearing age.

- **Position:** Place the patient in a seated position with the foot in a true lateral position. The intermalleolar line should be perpendicular to the film. The lateral aspect of the foot should be placed closest to the film.

- **Central Ray:** Perpendicular to the film and centered to the base of the third metatarsal.

- **Respiration:** Suspended expiration.

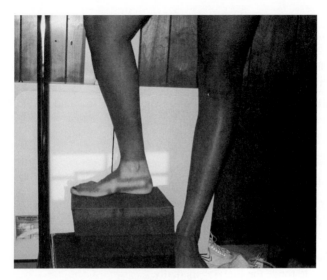

Figure 8–47. Lateral foot.

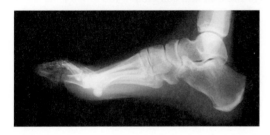

Figure 8–48. Lateral foot.

▶ MEDIAL OBLIQUE FOOT

- **Anatomy:** Phalanges, interphalangeal joints, metatarsals, cuboid, cuneiforms, navicular, and calcaneus.

- **Indication:** This is considered a basic view of the foot and should be performed with all foot series.

- **Film:** 10 × 12 in. crosswise without a grid.

- **Tube Tilt:** None.

- **FFD:** 40 in.

- **Safety:** Collimate to the soft tissue of the foot including toes. Gonadal shielding should be used on all children and on adults of childbearing age.

- **Position:** Place the patient in a seated or standing position. Instruct the patient to rotate the foot 45° medially.

- **Central Ray:** Perpendicular to the film and centered to the base of the third metatarsal.

- **Respiration:** Suspended expiration.

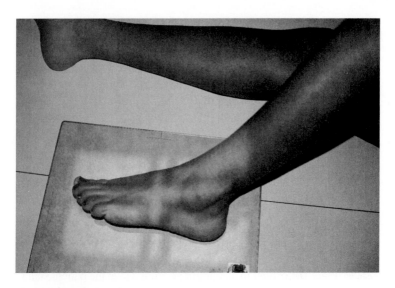

Figure 8–49. Medial oblique foot.

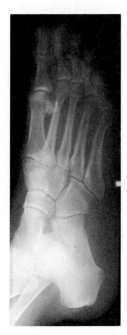

Figure 8–50. Medial oblique foot.

▶ LATERAL WEIGHT BEARING FOOT

- **Anatomy:** Calcaneus, talus, phalanges, interphalangeal joints, metatarsals, and tarsal bones.

- **Indication:** This view is performed in order to evaluate the arch of the foot with the patient in a full weight bearing position.

- **Film:** 10 × 12 crosswise without a grid. The film should be divided in half for two views.

- **Tube Tilt:** None.

- **FFD:** 40 in.

- **Safety:** Collimate to the soft tissue of the foot including toes. Gonadal shielding should be used on all children and on adults of childbearing age.

- **Position:** Place the patient in an upright position. Have the patient stand on a sponge or a small platform in order to drop the film below the level of the arch of the foot. Instruct the patient to place the affected foot against the film.

- **Central Ray:** Perpendicular to the film and centered to the base of the third metatarsal.

- **Respiration:** Suspended expiration.

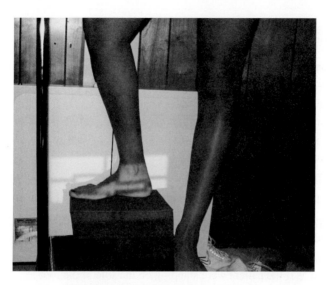

Figure 8–51. Lateral weight bearing foot.

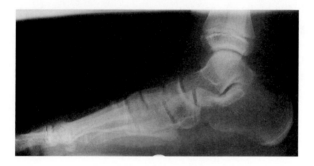

Figure 8–52. Lateral weight bearing foot.

▶ AP TOES

- **Anatomy:** Phalanges, interphalangeal joint spaces, metatarsophalangeal joint, and metatarsals.

- **Indication:** This is considered a basic view of the toes and should be performed with all toe series.

- **Film:** 8 × 10 in. crosswise without a grid. The film should be divided in thirds for three views.

- **Tube Tilt:** None.

- **FFD:** 40 in.

- **Safety:** Collimate to the soft tissue of the toe being x-rayed. Gonadal shielding should be used on children and on adults of childbearing age.

- **Position:** Place the patient in a seated or upright position with the foot placed as if the patient were standing on the sole of the foot.

- **Central Ray:** Perpendicular to the film and centered to the metatarsophalangeal joint of the affected toe.

- **Respiration:** Suspended expiration.

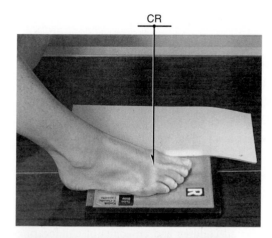

Figure 8–53. AP toes.

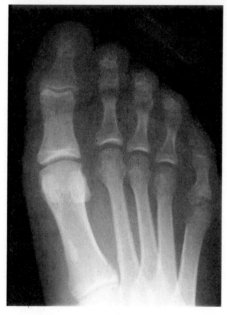

Figure 8–54. AP toes.

▶ LATERAL TOES

- **Anatomy:** Phalanges, interphalangeal joints, metatarsophalangeal joints, and metatarsals.

- **Indication:** This is considered a basic view of the toes and should be performed with all toe series.

- **Film:** 8 × 10 in. crosswise without a grid. The film should be divided into thirds for three views.

- **Tube Tilt:** None.

- **FFD:** 40 in.

- **Safety:** Collimate to the soft tissue of the toe being x-rayed. Gonadal shielding should be used on all children and on adults of childbearing age.

- **Position:** Place the patient in a seated position with the affected toe placed in a true lateral position. The medial aspect of the second and third digits should be placed closest to the film and the lateral aspect of the fourth and fifth digits should be placed closest to the film. Tape or gauze may be used to move the unaffected toes out the way to avoid superimposition.

- **Central Ray:** Perpendicular to the film and centered to the proximal interphalangeal joint space for the second through the fifth digits and the interphalangeal joint space for the first digit.

- **Respiration:** Suspended expiration.

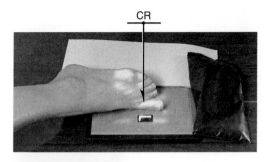

Figure 8–55. Lateral toes (first digit).

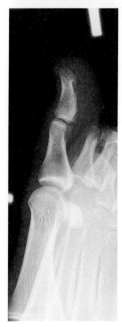

Figure 8–56. Lateral toes (first digit).

▶ OBLIQUE TOES

- **Anatomy:** Phalanges, interphalangeal joint spaces, metatarsophalangeal joint spaces, and metatarsals.

- **Indication:** This is considered a basic view of the toes and should be performed with all toe series.

- **Film:** 8 × 10 in. crosswise without a grid. The film should be divided in thirds for three views.

- **Tube Tilt:** None.

- **FFD:** 40 in.

- **Safety:** Collimate to the soft tissue of the toe being x-rayed. Gonadal shielding should be used on all children and on adults of childbearing age.

- **Position:** Place the patient in a seated position with the foot at a 45° angle. The foot should be positioned medially for the first, second, and third digits and laterally for the fourth and fifth digits.

- **Central Ray:** Perpendicular to the film and centered to the metatarsophalangeal joint of the affected digit.

- **Respiration:** Suspended expiration.

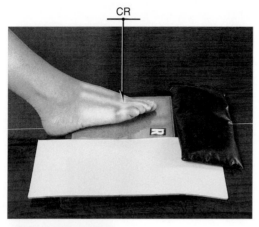

Figure 8–57. Oblique toes.

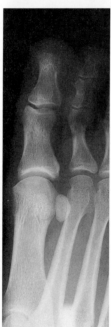

Figure 8–58. Oblique toes.

HEAD RADIOGRAPHY

9

► AP/PA SKULL

- **Anatomy:** Ethmoid sinus, frontal sinus, maxillary sinus, superior and inferior orbital shadows, and petrous ridges.

- **Indication:** This is considered a basic view of the skull and should be performed with all skull series. If an abnormality is present, then special imaging may be indicated.

- **Film:** 10 × 12 in. lengthwise with a grid.

- **Tube Tilt:** None.

- **FFD:** 40 in.

- **Safety:** Collimate to an area slightly less than the size of film being used. Gonadal shielding should be used on all children and on adults of childbearing age.

- **Position:** Place the patient in an upright position with the back against the Bucky for the AP position. For the PA position, the patient should be facing the Bucky. Place the head so that the orbitomeatal line (imaginary line between the eyes) is perpendicular to the film. This view may be done with the patient recumbent.

- **Central Ray:** Perpendicular to the film and centered to the nasion. For the PA projection, the central ray should be perpendicular to the Bucky and centered to exit through the nasion.

- **Respiration:** Suspended expiration.

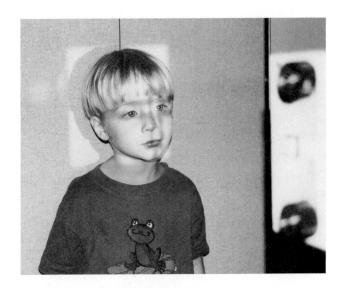

Figure 9–1. AP skull.

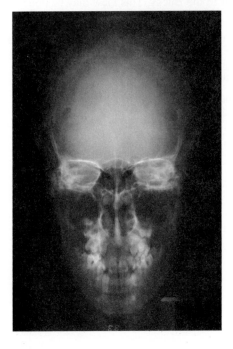

Figure 9–2. AP skull.

► LATERAL SKULL

- **Anatomy:** Sella turcica, anterior clinoid process, and posterior clinoid process.

- **Indication:** This is considered a basic view of the skull and should be performed with all skull series. If an abnormality is present, then special imaging may be indicated.

- **Film:** 10 × 12 in. crosswise with a grid.

- **Tube Tilt:** None.

- **FFD:** 40 in.

- **Safety:** Collimate to an area slightly less than the film being used. Gonadal shielding should be used on all children and on adults of childbearing age.

- **Position:** Place the patient in an upright position facing the Bucky. Instruct the patient to turn the head to a true lateral position. The interpupillary line should be perpendicular to the Bucky. This view may be done with the patient recumbent.

- **Central Ray:** Perpendicular to the film and centered 2 in. superior to the external auditory meatus.

- **Respiration:** Suspended expiration.

- **Notes:** The side of interest should be placed closest to the Bucky.

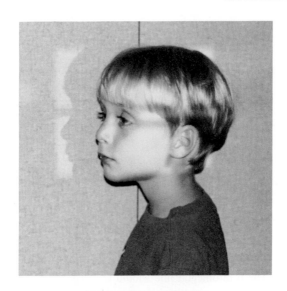

Figure 9–3. Lateral skull.

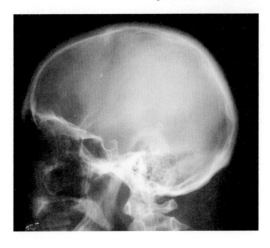

Figure 9–4. Lateral skull.

▶ AP AXIAL SKULL—TOWNE'S VIEW

- **Anatomy:** With a 30° tube tilt, the posterior clenoid processes, foramen magnum, dorsum sella, and petrous ridges are visualized. With a 37° caudal tube tilt, the anterior clenoid processes will also be visualized.

- **Indication:** This is considered a basic view and should be performed with all skull series.

- **Film:** 10 × 12 in. lengthwise with a grid.

- **Tube Tilt:** 30° to 37° caudad, depending on anatomy of interest.

- **FFD:** 40 in.

- **Safety:** Collimate to an area slightly less than the film being used. Gonadal shielding should be used on children and on adults of childbearing age.

- **Position:** Place the patient in the upright position with the back against the Bucky. The orbitomeatal line should be perpendicular to the film. This view may be done with the patient supine.

- **Central Ray:** If the dorsum, sella turcica, and posterior glenoid processes are of primary interest, the central ray should be 37° caudad and centered 1.5 in. superior to the supraciliary arch. If the anterior glenoid processes are of primary interest, the central ray should be 30° caudad and centered 1.5 in. superior to the supraciliary arch.

- **Respiration:** Suspended expiration.

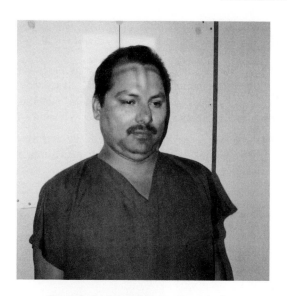

Figure 9–5. AP axial skull—Towne's view.

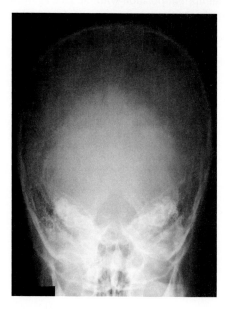

Figure 9–6. AP axial skull
—Towne's view.

► PA CALDWELL SKULL

- **Anatomy:** This view places the petrous ridges in the lower one-third of the orbits so that the superior orbital margin is visualized without superimposition. Also visualized are frontal sinuses, ethmoid sinuses, orbital margins, greater sphenoid wings, and lesser sphenoid wings.

- **Indication:** This is a basic view and should be performed with all skull series. If an abnormality is present, then special imaging may be indicated.

- **Film:** 10 × 12 in. lengthwise with a grid.

- **Tube Tilt:** 15° caudad.

- **FFD:** 40 in.

- **Safety:** Collimate to an area slightly less than the film being used. Gonadal shielding should be used on all children and on adults of childbearing age.

- **Position:** Place the patient in an upright position with the face against the Bucky. The orbitomeatal line should be placed perpendicular to the film.

- **Central Ray:** 15° caudad and centered to exit the nasion.

- **Respiration:** Suspended expiration.

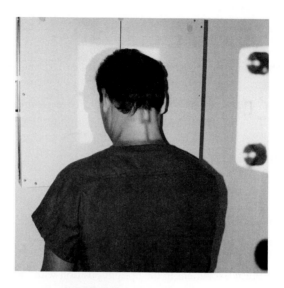

Figure 9–7. PA Caldwell skull.

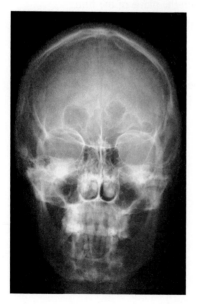

Figure 9–8. PA Caldwell skull.

▶ WATER'S VIEW OF THE SINUSES

- **Anatomy:** Frontal sinuses, ethmoid sinuses, maxillary sinuses, and foramen rotundum.

- **Indication:** This is a basic view and should be performed with all sinus series. If an abnormality is present, then special imaging may be indicated.

- **Film:** 10 × 12 in. lengthwise with a grid.

- **Tube Tilt:** None.

- **FFD:** 40 in.

- **Safety:** Collimate to an area slightly less than the film being used. Gonadal shielding should be used on all children and on adults of childbearing age.

- **Position:** Place the patient in the upright position with the face against the Bucky. Instruct the patient to rest the chin on the Bucky so that the orbitomeatal line forms a 37° angle with the plane of the film.

- **Central Ray:** Perpendicular to the film and centered to the vertex of the skull.

- **Respiration:** Suspended expiration.

- **Notes:** All sinus views should be performed with the patient in the upright position to visualize air/fluid levels.

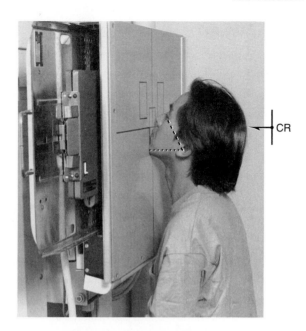

Figure 9–9. Water's view of the sinuses.

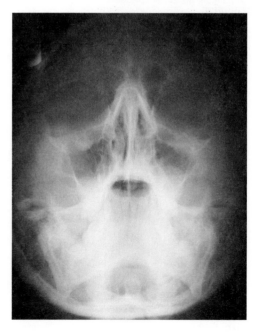

Figure 9–10. Water's view of the sinuses.

► LATERAL SINUSES

- **Anatomy:** Frontal sinuses, maxillary sinuses, and sphenoid sinuses.

- **Indication:** This is considered a basic view and should be performed with all sinus series. If an abnormality is present, special imaging may be indicated.

- **Film:** 10 × 12 in. crosswise with a grid.

- **Tube Tilt:** None.

- **FFD:** 40 in.

- **Safety:** Collimate to an area slightly less than the film being used. Gonadal shielding should be used on all children and on adults of childbearing age.

- **Position:** Place the patient in an upright position with the face against the Bucky. Place the side of interest closest to the film with the interpupillary line perpendicular to the film.

- **Central Ray:** Perpendicular to the film and centered 0.5 to 1 in. posterior to the outer canthus of the eye.

- **Respiration:** Suspended expiration.

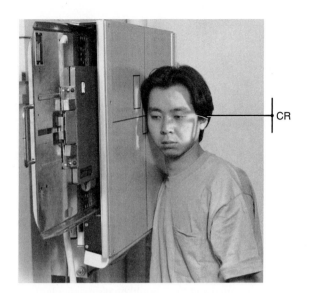

Figure 9–11. Lateral sinuses.

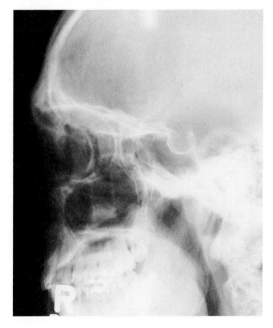

Figure 9–12. Lateral sinuses.

► PA CALDWELL SINUSES

- **Anatomy:** Frontal sinuses, ethmoid sinuses, sphenoid sinuses, maxillary sinuses, and petrous ridges in the lower one-third of the orbits.

- **Indication:** This is considered a basic view and should be performed with all sinus series. If an abnormality is present, then special imaging may be indicated.

- **Film:** 10 × 12 in. lengthwise with a grid.

- **Tube Tilt:** 15° caudad.

- **FFD:** 40 in.

- **Safety:** Collimate to an area slightly less than the film being used. Gonadal shielding should be used on all children and on adults of childbearing age.

- **Position:** Place the patient in an upright position with the face against the Bucky. The orbitomeatal line should be perpendicular to the Bucky.

- **Central Ray:** 15° caudad and centered to exit through the nasion.

- **Respiration:** Suspended expiration.

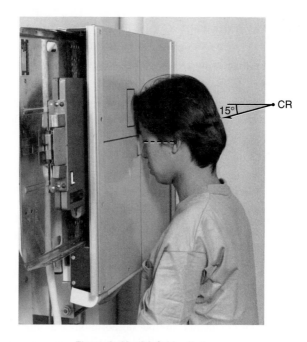

Figure 9–13. PA Caldwell sinuses.

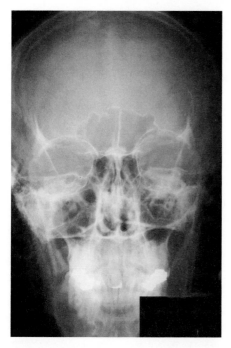

Figure 9–14. PA Caldwell sinuses.

▶ SUBMENTOVERTEX SINUSES

- **Anatomy:** Maxillary sinuses, ethmoid sinuses, vomer, sphenoid sinuses, and clivus.

- **Indication:** This is considered a basic view and should be performed with all sinus series. If an abnormality is present, then special imaging may be indicated.

- **Film:** 10 × 12 in. lengthwise with a grid.

- **Tube Tilt:** None.

- **FFD:** 40 in.

- **Safety:** Collimate to an area slightly less than the film being used. Gonadal shielding should be used on all children and on adults of childbearing age.

- **Position:** Place the patient in an upright position with the back against the Bucky. Instruct the patient to hyperextend the neck so the infraorbitomeatal line is parallel to the Bucky.

- **Central Ray:** Perpendicular to the infraorbitomeatal line and centered between the angles of the mandible and 0.75 in. anterior to the external auditory meatus.

- **Respiration:** Suspended expiration.

- **Notes:** If the patient is unable to place the head so that the infraorbitomeatal line is parallel to the film, then a tube tilt may be required to place it perpendicular to the infraorbital meatal line.

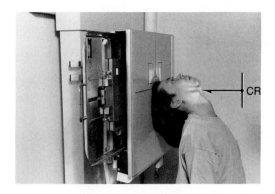

Figure 9–15. Submentovertex sinuses.

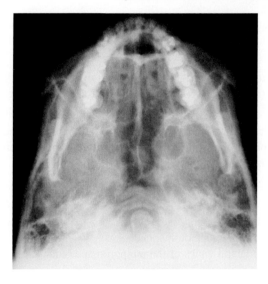

Figure 9–16. Submento-vertex sinuses.

▶ LATERAL AXIAL TEMPOROMANDIBULAR JOINT— LAW METHOD

- **Anatomy:** Temporomandibular joint (TMJ) closest to the Bucky. This view is performed with the patient's mouth open and closed to demonstrate the position of the condyles in both positions.

- **Indication:** This is considered a basic view and should be performed with all temporomandibular joint series.

- **Film:** 8 × 10 in. crosswise with a grid.

- **Tube Tilt:** 15° caudad.

- **FFD:** 40 in.

- **Safety:** Collimate to an area slightly less than the film being used. Gonadal shielding should be used on all children and on adults of childbearing age.

- **Position:** Place the patient in an upright position with the face against the Bucky. Place the patient in a true lateral position and then rotate the head towards the film 15°. This view may be done with the patient recumbent.

- **Central Ray:** 15° caudad and centered 1.5 in. superior to the external auditory meatus. This places the central ray exiting through the temporomandibular joint closest to the Bucky.

- **Respiration:** Suspended expiration.

- **Notes:**
  1. This view should be performed with the patient's mouth closed and then again with the patient's mouth opened.
  2. Always perform bilateral views of the temporomandibular joints for comparison.

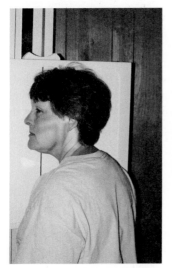
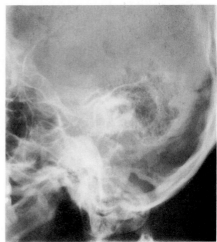

Figure 9–17. Lateral axial temporomandibular joint—Law method. Closed mouth.

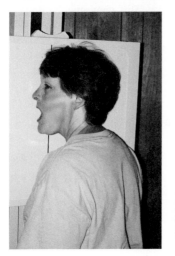
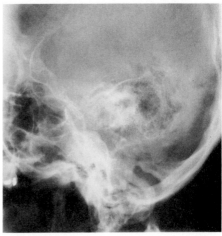

Figure 9–18. Lateral axial temporomandibular joint—Law method. Open mouth.

► LATERAL AXIAL TEMPORMANDIBULAR JOINTS— SCHULLER METHOD

- **Anatomy:** Temporomandibular joint closest to the Bucky. Always do bilateral views of the temporomandibular joints with the patient's mouth opened and closed to compare the position of the condyles bilaterally.

- **Indication:** This is considered a basic view and should be performed with all TMJ series.

- **Film:** 8 × 10 in. crosswise with a grid.

- **Tube Tilt:** 25° to 30° caudad.

- **FFD:** 40 in.

- **Safety:** Collimate to an area slightly less than the film being used. Gonadal shielding should be used on children and on adults of childbearing age.

- **Position:** Place the patient in an upright position with the face against the Bucky. Place the patient's head in a true lateral position with the interpupillary line perpendicular to the Bucky. This view may be done with the patient recumbent.

- **Central Ray:** 25° to 30° caudad and centered 0.5 in. anterior and 2 in. superior to the external auditory meatus.

- **Respiration:** Suspended expiration.

- **Notes:**
  1. This view should be performed with the patient's mouth opened and closed.
  2. Always perform bilateral views of the temporomandibular joints for comparison.

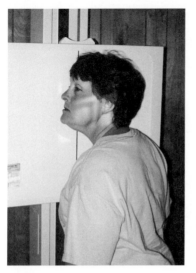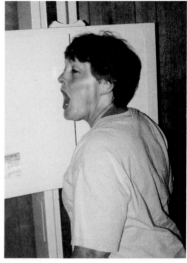

Figure 9–19. Lateral axial temporomandibular joint—Schuller method. **A.** Closed mouth. **B.** Open mouth.

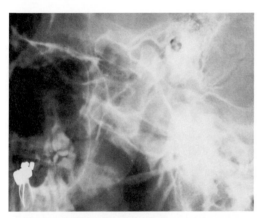

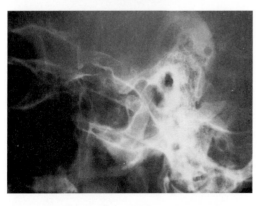

Figure 9–20. Lateral axial temporomandibular joint—Schuller method. **A.** Closed mouth. **B.** Open mouth.

CHEST AND ABDOMINAL RADIOGRAPHY

► PA CHEST

- **Anatomy:** Clavicles, ribs, apices of the lungs, aortic arch, heart, hilar regions, thoracic vertebrae, right and left costophrenic angles, and right and left hemidiaphragms.

- **Indication:** This is considered a basic view and should be performed with all chest series. If an abnormality is present, special imaging may be indicated.

- **Film:** 14 × 17 in. lengthwise with a grid.

- **Tube Tilt:** None.

- **FFD:** 72 in. (All chest x-rays should be performed at 72 in. to decrease magnification of the heart.)

- **Safety:** Collimate to an area slightly less than the film being used. Gonadal shielding should be used on all children and on adults of childbearing age.

- **Position:** Place the patient in an upright position with the chest against the Bucky. Instruct the patient to elevate the chin, roll the shoulders toward the Bucky, and depress the shoulders downward.

- **Central Ray:** Perpendicular to the film and centered to T7.

- **Respiration:** Full inspiration.

- **Notes:**
  1. It is very important to have the patient roll the shoulders forward to avoid superimposition of the scapulae in the lung fields.
  2. Always perform chest x-rays on full inspiration to fill the lungs with air as much as possible.

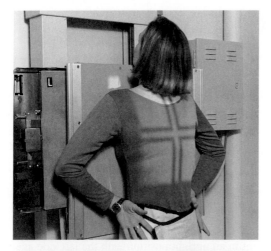

Figure 10–1. PA chest.

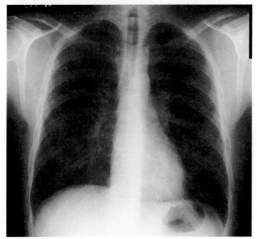

Figure 10–2. PA chest.

▶ LATERAL CHEST

- **Anatomy:** Thoracic vertebrae, hilae, heart, diaphragms, and costophrenic angles.

- **Indication:** This is considered a basic view and should be performed with all chest series. If an abnormality is present, then special imaging may be indicated.

- **Film:** 14 × 17 in. lengthwise with a grid.

- **FFD:** 72 in.

- **Safety:** Collimate to an area slightly less than the film being used. Gonadal shielding should be used on all children and on adults of childbearing age.

- **Position:** Place the patient in an upright position with the left side against the Bucky. Instruct the patient to elevate the arms above the head. Make sure the patient's pelvis and shoulders are in a true lateral position.

- **Central Ray:** Perpendicular to the film and centered to T7.

- **Respiration:** Full inspiration.

- **Notes:** Lateral chest x-rays are always done with the left side closest to the film to decrease magnification of the heart unless otherwise indicated.

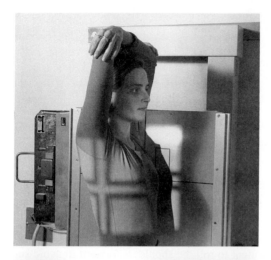

Figure 10–3. Lateral chest.

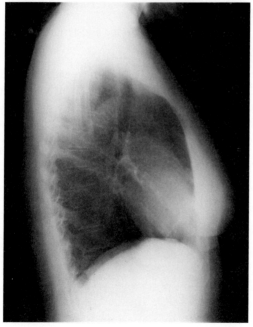

Figure 10–4. Lateral chest.

► APICAL LORDOTIC CHEST

- **Anatomy:** Apices of the lungs, clavicles, and ribs.

- **Indication:** This view should be performed when a tumor of the apical region is suspected.

- **Film:** 14 × 17 in. lengthwise with a grid.

- **Tube Tilt:** 15° to 20° cephalad.

- **FFD:** 72 in.

- **Safety:** Collimate to an area slightly less than the film being used. Gonadal shielding should be used on all children and on adults of childbearing age.

- **Position:** Place the patient in an upright position with the back against the Bucky. Instruct the patient to roll the shoulders forward to avoid superimposition of the scapulae in the lung fields.

- **Central Ray:** 15° to 20° cephalad and centered to the midsternum region.

- **Respiration:** Suspended inspiration.

- **Notes:** If the patient is able, this view may be performed with no tube tilt and with the patient leaning back against the Bucky. If this view is preferred, place the patient approximately 1 ft. from the Bucky and instruct the patient to lean back with the shoulders, neck, and back of head against the Bucky.

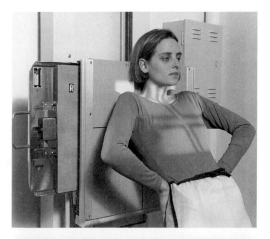

Figure 10–5. Apical lordotic chest.

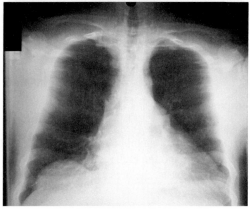

Figure 10–6. Apical lordotic chest.

► LATERAL STERNUM

- **Anatomy:** Manubrium, sternal angle, body, and xyphoid process.
- **Indication:** This view is considered a basic view and should be performed with all sternal series.
- **Film:** 10 × 12 in. lengthwise with a grid.
- **Tube Tilt:** None.
- **FFD:** 40 in. (A 72-in. FFD may be used to reduce magnification of the sternum.)
- **Safety:** Collimate to the soft tissue of the sternum. Gonadal shielding should be used on children and on adults of childbearing age.
- **Position:** Place the patient in an upright position with the left side against the Bucky. Place the shoulders posterior by locking the hands behind the back. (This will project the sternum forward.) This view may be done with the patient recumbent.
- **Central Ray:** Perpendicular to the film and centered to the midsternal region.
- **Respiration:** Suspended inspiration.
- **Notes:**
  1. This is performed on inspiration to obtain better contrast between the posterior aspect of the sternum and the lung region.
  2. If a female patient has large breasts, the breasts may be placed to the side by using a wide bandage.

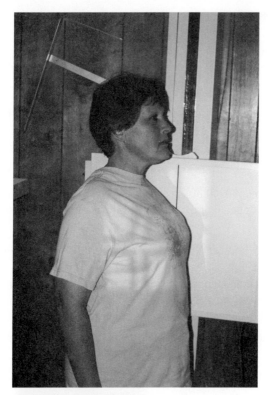

Figure 10–7. Lateral sternum.

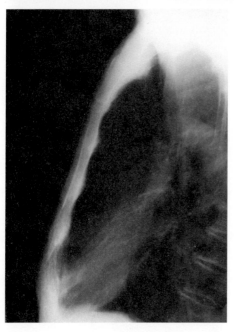

Figure 10–8. Lateral sternum.

▶ RIGHT ANTERIOR OBLIQUE STERNUM

- **Anatomy:** Manubrium, body, xyphoid process, and sternal angle.

- **Indication:** This is considered a basic view and should be performed with all sternal series.

- **Film:** 10 × 12 in. lengthwise with a grid.

- **Tube Tilt:** None.

- **FFD:** As short as possible (30–40 in.). A shorter FFD causes magnification of the sternum and loses detail of the surrounding anatomy to better visualize the sternum.

- **Safety:** Collimate to the soft tissue of the sternum. Gonadal shielding should be used on all children and on adults of childbearing age.

- **Position:** Place the patient in an upright position with the chest against the Bucky. Placing the patient in a right anterior oblique (15° to 20°) position. This view may be done with the patient recumbent.

- **Central Ray:** Perpendicular to the film and centered to the midsternal region.

- **Respiration:** Suspended expiration.

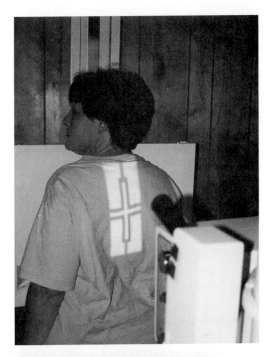

Figure 10–9. RAO sternum.

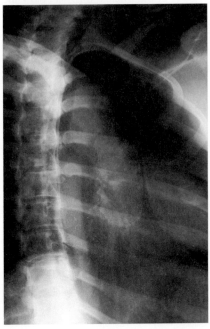

Figure 10–10. RAO sternum.

► AP/PA RIBS ABOVE AND BELOW THE DIAPHRAGM

- **Anatomy:** Ribs, clavicle, and heart shadow.

- **Indication:** This is considered a basic view and should be performed with all rib series.

- **Film:** 14 × 17 in. crosswise with a grid.

- **Tube Tilt:** None.

- **FFD:** 40 in.

- **Safety:** Collimate to an area slightly less than the film being used. Gonadal shielding should be used on all children and on adults of childbearing age.

- **Position:** Place the patient in an upright position with the back against the Bucky when the posterior ribs are of primary interest. Place the patient in an upright position with the chest against the Bucky when the anterior ribs are of primary interest. These views may be done with the patient recumbent.

- **Central Ray:** Perpendicular to the Bucky and centered to the level of T7 for ribs above the diaphragm and centered to a level halfway between the xyphoid process and the lower edge of the ribcage for ribs below the diaphragm.

- **Respiration:** For ribs above the diaphragm, suspended inspiration in order to move the lower diaphragm out of the way. For ribs below the diaphragm, suspended expiration to raise the diaphragm out of the way.

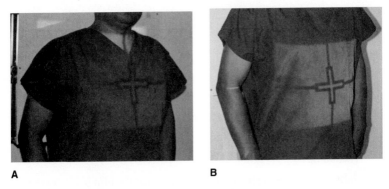

Figure 10–11. A. AP ribs above the diaphragm. **B.** AP ribs below the diaphragm.

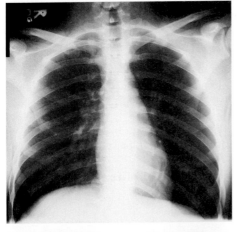

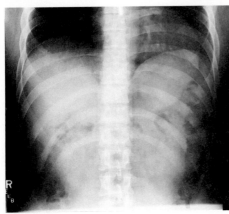

Figure 10–12. A. AP ribs above the diaphragm. **B.** AP ribs below the diaphragm.

▶ ANTERIOR AND POSTERIOR OBLIQUE RIBS

- **Anatomy:** Axillary margins of the ribs.

- **Indication:** This is considered a basic view of the ribs and should be performed with all rib series.

- **Film:** 14 × 17 in. lengthwise with a grid.

- **Tube Tilt:** None.

- **FFD:** 40 in.

- **Safety:** Collimate to an area slightly less than the film being used. Gonadal shielding should be used on all children and on adults of childbearing age.

- **Position:** Place the patient in an upright position with the body rotated 45° into a posterior or anterior oblique position. These views may be done with the patient recumbent.

- **Central Ray:** Perpendicular to the Bucky and centered midway between the lateral margin of the ribs and the spine and centered to the film.

- **Respiration:** Suspended expiration.

- **Notes:**
  1. For posterior obliques (RPO/LPO), place the affected side closest to the Bucky.
  2. For anterior obliques (RAO/LAO), place the affected side away from the Bucky.

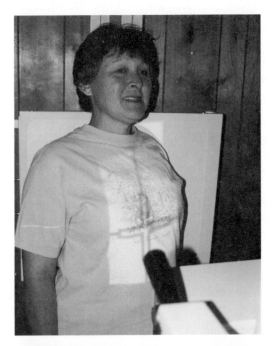

Figure 10–13. RPO ribs.

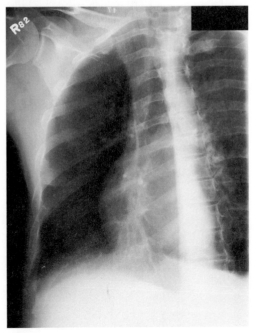

Figure 10–14. RPO ribs.

► AP ABDOMEN—SUPINE

- **Anatomy:** Liver, kidneys, psoas muscle, lumbar spine, pelvis, lower ribs, and bowel gas patterns.

- **Indication:** This is considered a basic view and should be performed with all abdomen series.

- **Film:** 14 × 17 in. lengthwise with a grid.

- **Tube Tilt:** None.

- **FFD:** 40 in.

- **Safety:** Collimate to the soft tissue of the abdomen crosswise and slightly less than the length of film being used. Gonadal shielding should be used on all children and on adults if possible with the anatomy being obscured.

- **Position:** Place the patient in a supine position with the back against the Bucky.

- **Central Ray:** Perpendicular to the film and centered to the level of the iliac crest.

- **Respiration:** Suspended expiration.

- **Notes:** This view may be referred to as a KUB, which stands for kidneys, ureters, and bladder; these organs should be included on the film.

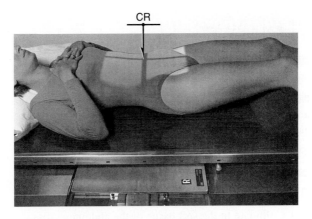

Figure 10–15. AP abdomen—supine.

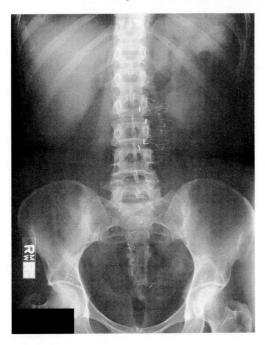

Figure 10–16. AP abdomen
—supine.

▶ AP ABDOMEN—ERECT

- **Anatomy:** Diaphragm, liver, kidneys, lumbar spine, lower ribs, pelvis, and bowel gas and air fluid levels.

- **Indication:** This view is specifically performed to evaluate air fluid levels of the abdomen in the case of a possible small bowel obstruction or perforated bowel.

- **Film:** 14 × 17 in. lengthwise with a grid.

- **Tube Tilt:** None.

- **FFD:** 40 in.

- **Safety:** Collimate to the soft tissue of the abdomen crosswise and slightly less than the length of film being used. Gonadal shielding should be used on all children and on adults when possible without the anatomy being obscured.

- **Position:** Place the patient in an upright position with the back against the Bucky. Make sure there is no rotation of the pelvis or shoulders.

- **Central Ray:** Perpendicular to the Bucky and centered 1–2 in. above the level of the iliac crest.

- **Respiration:** Suspended expiration.

- **Notes:** Make sure the diaphragm is included, in order to evaluate free air under the diaphragm.

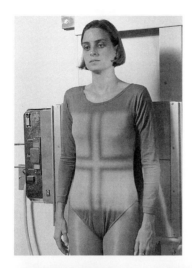

Figure 10–17. AP abdomen
—erect.

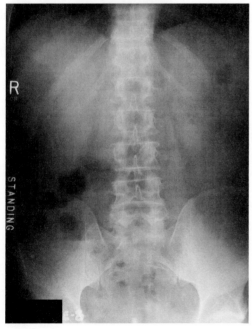

Figure 10–18. AP abdomen
—erect.

PRINCIPLES OF
ADVANCED IMAGING

Lawrence H. Wyatt, D.C., D.A.C.B.R.

COMPUTED TOMOGRAPHY

Computed tomography (CT) scanning is an advanced imaging procedure that uses conventional x-radiation to produce axial and reconstructed images in any plane of the human body with the use of a thin fan-shaped x-ray beam.

Image Acquisition

- Carefully collimated fan-shaped x-ray beam penetrates patient.
- X-ray beam width is equal to "slice thickness" desired, typically 1–10 mm.
- X-ray beam rotates around patient in a 180° arc.
- Radiation detectors measure the radiation that has passed through the patient.
- Computer correlates:
  - Patient location inside scanner gantry.
  - Relationship of x-ray beam to area being imaged.
  - Intensity of radiation passing through the patient.
- Images can be reconstructed in any plane by computer manipulation.

Images

Figures 11–1 and 11–2 are normal CT scans of the cervical and lumbar spine.

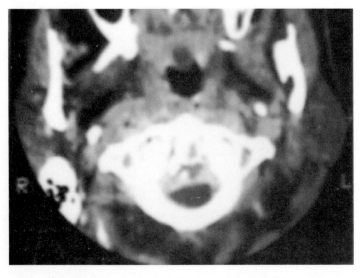

Figure 11–1. Normal CT scan of cervical spine.

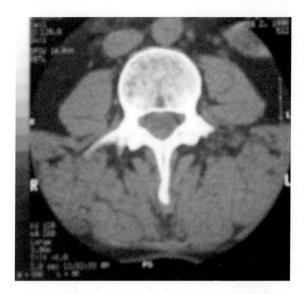

Figure 11–2. Normal CT scan of lumbar spine.

Advantages

- Contrast resolution is over 95 times better than conventional radiography.
- Three-dimensional images can be made in any plane of the body.
- No film-based imaging receptor.
- Window/level settings can be used to highlight bone or soft tissue.
- Tissue densities can be quantified with Hounsfield unit measurement (Table 11–1).

Limitations

- Motion artifacts can be caused by patient movement during scanning.
- Beam-hardening artifacts can be caused by metal or thick bone concentration (such as in the posterior skull base).

TABLE 11–1. NORMAL HOUNSFIELD CT NUMBERS FOR HUMAN TISSUES

Tissue	CT Number
Air	−1000
Fat	−100
Water	0
CSF	15
Blood	40
Cortical bone	+1000

- Size limitations of gantry and table prohibit imaging very large patients.
- Reconstructed images are not particularly sharp.

Indications
- Abdominal masses
- Cauda equina syndrome
- Cerebral masses
- Cerebral ischemia
- Disc protrusion/extrusion/prolapse
- Headache of unknown etiology
- Intracanilicular masses
- Follow-up of unusual plain film findings (e.g., suspected fracture)

Contraindications
- Very large patients
- Pregnancy (clinical decision left to physician based on threat to mother's life).

Patient Preparation
- Normally none.
- If contrast used (e.g., head, abdomen, chest), consult with radiologist.

MAGNETIC RESONANCE IMAGING
Magnetic resonance imaging (MRI) involves the use of the inherent magnetism inside the body and radio frequency waves to produce images of the body in any plane necessary.

Image Acquisition
- Patient placed inside a large magnetic field (magnet inside gantry).
- Radio frequency wave introduced causes H^+ atoms to change orientation.
- Radio frequency wave removed causes H^+ atoms to return to normal position.
- Radio frequency waves are given off as they return to position.
- Detectors measure energy given off during repositioning.
- Computer correlates:
  - Patient location inside gantry.
  - Relationship of radio frequency energy to area being imaged.
  - Intensity of radio frequency energy.
  - Speed of return of radio frequency energy to detectors (T1/T2 relaxation times).

Images
Figures 11–3 to 11–6 are normal T1- and T2-weighted MRI scans of the cervical and lumbar spine. T1-weighted images highlight fatty tissues as the

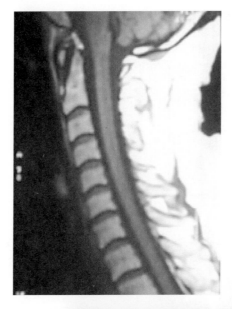

Figure 11–3. T1-weighted MRI scan of cervical spine.

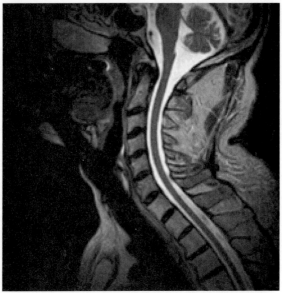

Figure 11–4. T2-weighted MRI scan of cervical spine.

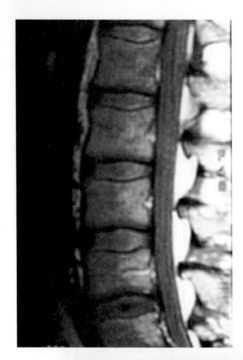

Figure 11–5. T1-weighted MRI scan of lumbar spine.

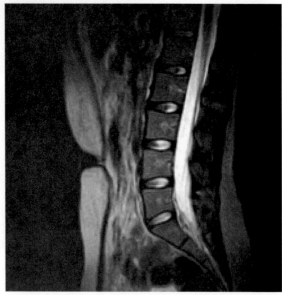

Figure 11–6. T2-weighted MRI scan of lumbar spine.

brightest signal intensity. T2-weighted images highlight water-based tissues (e.g., CSF) as the brightest signal.

Advantages
- Very high soft tissue contrast and spatial resolution.
- No x-radiation.
- No known adverse biologic effects.

Limitations
- Patient size limited by gantry size.
- Patients with ferromagnetic implants often cannot be imaged.
- Patients must remain motionless for long periods of time.
- Patients can become claustrophobic inside gantry.

Indications
- Spinal cord pathology
- Disc disease
- Nonacute intracranial lesions.
- Solid organ abdominal pathology (e.g., liver)
- Marrow replacement disorders (metastasis)
- Demyelinating CNS disorders
- Musculotendinous disorders

Contraindications
- Ferromagnetic joint prostheses
- Pacemakers
- Implanted cardiac defibrillators
- Intracranial aneurysm clips
- Surgical clips
- Metallic foreign bodies (e.g., shrapnel)
- Implanted CNS stimulators
- Metallic prosthetic heart valves
- Cochlear implants

Patient Preparation
- Normally none.
- If contrast will be used (e.g., head, abdomen, chest), consult with radiologist.
- No makeup.
- Inform radiologist of claustrophobia.

RADIONUCLIDE BONE IMAGING
Radionuclide bone imaging (bone scan) involves the use of radioactive pharmaceuticals injected into the patient to determine any significant localized or

systemic increase or decrease in osseous metabolic activity associated with bone disease.

Image Acquisition

- Commonly used radiopharmaceuticals are technetium 99m phosphate compounds and indium 111-labeled white blood cells.
- Patient injected with radiopharmaceutical.
- Sequential images are obtained every 3 seconds for 60 seconds over area of concern.
- Immediately after flow study, blood pool images are obtained over area of concern.
- After at least 2 hours, multiple images are obtained over entire skeleton.
- Spot images can also be obtained.

Images

Figures 11–7A and 11–7B demonstrate normal anterior and posterior full-skeleton static images. There are certain areas of the body that have normally increased uptake of the radiopharmaceutical (Table 11–2).

Advantages

- Highly sensitive (can detect 2–3% bone loss).
- Bones are well seen with minimal soft tissue uptake.
- Defines entire skeleton on one image.

Limitations

- Patient rotation can have profound effect on images, creating false positives.
- Urine retained in lower renal calyx may overylay lower rib(s).
- Jewelry creates cold defects.
- Breast prostheses can give asymmetrical activity over chest.
- Recent dental procedures may create increased uptake in jaws.
- Poor specificity.

Indications

- Primary bone tumors
- Metastasis
- Osteomyelitis
- Avascular necrosis of bone
- Occult fractures
- Stress fractures

Contraindications

- Pregnancy

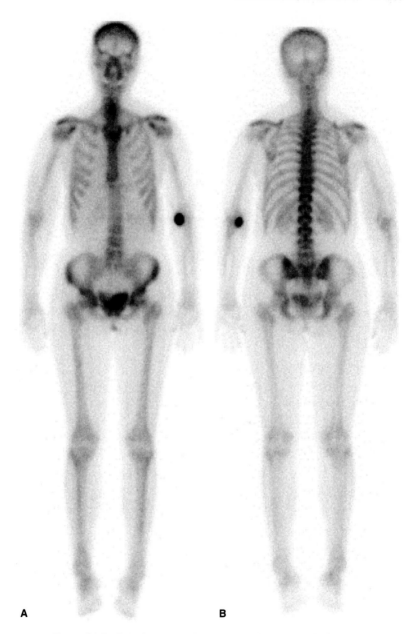

Figure 11–7. Full-skeleton static bone scan. **A.** Anterior. **B.** Posterior.

TABLE 11–2. NORMAL AREAS OF INCREASED UPTAKE ON BONE SCANS

Sacroiliac joints
Kidneys
Acromioclavicular joints
Sternoclavicular joints
Tips of the scapulae
Costochondral junctions
Frontal parasagittal regions of the skull

Patient Preparation
- Good hydration prior to scanning.

DOPPLER ULTRASOUND
Doppler ultrasound involves the use of ultrasonic waves to detect blood flow abnormalities. It is most useful to chiropractors in the evaluation of carotid and vertebrobasilar vascular insufficiency. Modern scanners can image in color.

Image Acquisition
- Transducer used with continuous/pulsed wave ultrasound.
- Both transverse and longitudinal images are obtained.
- Computer analyzes the difference in frequency between the emitted and received frequencies.
- Blood flow images are produced by computer manipulation of these differences.

Images
Figure 11–8 shows part of a normal carotid artery Doppler ultrasound study.

Advantages
- Very sensitive imaging of blood flow.
- Noninvasive procedure (e.g., no x-radiation).

Limitations
- None.

Indications
- Carotid artery insufficiency.
- Vertebrobasilar insufficiency.

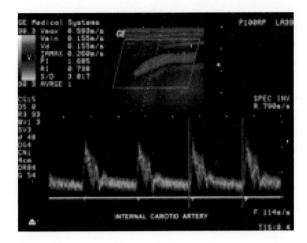

Figure 11–8. Normal carotid artery Doppler ultrasound image.

Patient Preparation

- Nothing in particular.
- Consult radiologist for specific instructions.

APPENDIXES

APPENDIX 1

Equipment Malfunction Guide

I. No Exposure
  A. No power to the generator
    • The machine is not turned on.
    • Circuit breaker is tripped.
  B. Control panel settings or switches engaged
    • Preparation button and exposure are not pushed simultaneously.
    • Incorrect bucky is chosen.
  C. Automatic collimator
    • Bucky is not pushed in completely.
    • FFD is not locked into specific distance.
    • Both the table and upright bucky are engaged, causing confusion to the control panel.
  D. Rotor operating but no exposure
    • Rotor may not be operating at correct speed to allow exposure to take place.
    • Selected filament may be burned out. (This is checked by using a different mA station to see whether an image is produced.)
II. Incorrect Radiographic Density
  A. Images are too light
    • Rare Earth cassette is upside down. (Yellow side of cassette acts as a low ratio grid.)
    • Mismatched film/screen combinations, such as light spectrum and speed.
    1. X-ray generator and x-ray tube
      • Timer circuits fail, having a shorter time of exposure than set on the control panel.
      • Control settings change without warning due to a power overload to the generator.
      • mA and kVp are miscallibrated. (This problem is picked up by a good quality control program.)
      • Filament is burning out. (Try using a different mA station.)

2. Darkroom and processing
   - Decrease in developer activity due to decreased temperature, decreased replenishment, improperly mixed developer, or low developer level.
   - Film is stopped in fixer for a longer period of time.
3. Ancillary equipment
   - Wrong grid. (A higher ratio of grid is used than expected.)
   - Grid cutoff. (Incorrect FFD, or central ray is not perpendicular to the grid.)
   - FFD is incorrect. (Longer FFD than expected.)

B. Images are too dark
   - Screen film speed is faster than technique chart allows for.
   - Cassettes with different density characteristics have been replaced with the same screens.

1. X-ray generator and x-ray tube
   - Timer circuits fail, giving more time than expected.
   - Changes in technical factors due to power surges.
   - Multi-exposures due to faulty exposure switch.
   - Miscallibration of the mA and/or kVp, which should be demonstrated through the quality control problem.
2. Darkroom and processing
   - Developer activity is increased due to increased temperature, overreplenishment, or improperly mixed developer.
   - Fogged films from light leaks, expiration of film, or exposure to excessive heat or radiation.
3. Ancillary equipment
   - Inappropriate grid ratio. (Lower grid ratio than expected.)
   - Inappropriate beam size allowing more scattered radiation to affect the film.
   - Less filtration in place than specified.
   - FFD is less than expected.

III. Unsharp Images
A. Motion
   - Patient movement.
   - Image receptor movement.
   - Tube stand movement.
B. Geometric blurring
   - Focal spot is larger than intended from overuse.
   - Object film distance is larger than normal.
C. Image receptor
   - Poor film screen contact due to warped cassettes.
   - Screen film speed is too fast.

IV. Low Contrast Images
   A. Technical factors
      - kVp is too high for the part or pathology being x-rayed.
      - Incorrect grid for the part. (Low grid ratio allows more scattered radiation to contact the film.)
   B. Processing
      - Developer activity is altered due to contamination, exhaustion, or low developer temperature.
      - Fixer exhaustion.
   C. Image receptor
      - Base plus fog is increased due to improper storage of the film or expired film.
      - Screen colored spectrum does not match the film.
V. Misalignment of the Part and Image Receptor
      - Bucky is not pushed in all the way.
      - Tube is not centered correctly to the table/bucky.
      - Tube may be angled.
      - Crossbar template on collimator is out of position.

APPENDIX 2

Sample Forms for Technical Control of Radiologic Suite

1. QUALITY CONTROL PROGRAM TROUBLESHOOTING GUIDE

Upon receipt of your Davenport computerized test results, please note if any of your parameters are not within those acceptability limits previously detailed.

If any of your results are unacceptable, refer to the following information:

If the FOG is TOO HIGH	CHECK A, B, C, D, E, F, G, H
If the CONTRAST is TOO LOW	CHECK A, H, B, F, G, E, C, D, I
If the CONTRAST is TOO HIGH	CHECK A, E
If the SPEED is TOO LOW	CHECK A, H, E, F, I
If the SPEED is TOO HIGH	CHECK A, F, B, G, E, D, C, I
If the films are WET	CHECK G, J, E, H
If the films are FOGGED	CHECK G
If the films are DIRTY	CHECK K, L, J
If the films are SCRATCHED	CHECK M, G, J, H, L

A	Developer Temperature
B	Starter Absence during Preparation
C	Darkroom Illumination
D	Film Storage
E	Incorrect Replenishment Rate
F	Fixer in Developer
G	Fixer Exhausted
H	Developer Exhausted
I	Insufficient Circulation
J	Dryer Problems
K	Dirty Chemicals
L	Dirty Rollers
M	Film Transport System

Courtesy of the Gilbert X-ray Company of Texas.

2. PROCESSOR CHEMICAL STANDARDS

Processor Make/Model #1: _____	*Chemicals Used:* _____
Developer Temperature: _____	*Dev Replen Rate:* _____ *cc*
Dryer Temperature: _____	*Fix Replen Rate:* _____ *cc*
Water Temperature: _____	*Starter Quantity:* _____
Developer Immersion Time: _____	*Date Standards Set:* _____

PREVENTIVE MAINTENANCE/CLEANING SCHEDULE...Unit #: ___

4 WEEKS: ☐   6 WEEKS: ☐   8 WEEKS: ☐   OTHER: ☐

Date of Last PM	*Engineer Name*	*Date of Last PM*	*Engineer Name*

Courtesy of the Gilbert X-ray Company of Texas.

3. ROUTINE COMPLIANCE TESTING CHECKLIST

Customer Name: _____ *Account #:* _____

Address: _____ *Phone #:* _____

Contact Name: _____ *Title:* _____

Equipment Manufacturer: _____ *Model #:* _____

Equipment Serial #: _____ *Location:* _____

Gilbert Field Service Engineer: _____
                                             Signature

Date of PM/Calibration: _____ *SR #:* _____

X-ray PM/Calibration on Room #: _____

1. Perform kVp, mA, and timer checks and record: YES ☐   NO ☐

2. Perform techniques overload protection tests: YES ☐   NO ☐

3. Check collimator sizing and alignment: YES ☐   NO ☐

4. Observe phototimer operation: YES ☐   NO ☐

5. Check mechanical condition of tubestand or overhead tube mount, including locks: YES ☐   NO ☐

6. Check all movements for smooth, full travel: YES ☐   NO ☐

7. Inspect and lubricate all aircraft cables, balance springs, belts, chains, and gears: YES ☐   NO ☐

8. Observe all table motion limits, accessories, and components: YES ☐   NO ☐

9. Inspect and check all electrical connectors: YES ☐   NO ☐

10. Inspect all motor driven components: YES ☐   NO ☐

11. Check HV wells and re-compound: YES ☐   NO ☐

12. Inspect controls for proper labels: YES ☐   NO ☐

13. Inspect all contactors: YES ☐   NO ☐

14. Inspect TV and image tube condition/operation: YES ☐   NO ☐

15. Review PM/Calibration with customer; record all needed repairs and review with customer: YES ☐   NO ☐

16. Verify that ALL PM/Calibration data has been recorded for each specific test: YES ☐   NO ☐

_____

Courtesy of the Gilbert X-ray Company of Texas.

4. FILM PROCESSING UNIT CHECKLIST

Customer Name: _____ Account #: _____

Address: _____ Phone #: _____

Equipment Manufacturer: _____ Model #: _____

Location of processor: _____ Date of PM: _____

Gilbert Field Service Engineer: _____

1. Remove front, sides, cover and clean as needed:	YES ☐	NO ☐
2. Check temperature of developer, wash, and dryer:	YES ☐	NO ☐
3. Examine all tubing and connections:	YES ☐	NO ☐
4. Clean tanks of chemical deposits, build-up on support bars, shafts, gears, and drive chains:	YES ☐	NO ☐
5. Clean area around tanks:	YES ☐	NO ☐
6. Check dryer section for debris on rollers, wear of belt and pulleys, clean air tubes:	YES ☐	NO ☐
7. Clean all spills from underside and check all replenishment lines and screens:	YES ☐	NO ☐
8. Replace all filters if necessary:	YES ☐	NO ☐
9. Rinse tanks and flush recirculation lines:	YES ☐	NO ☐
10. Close drain lines and refill processor with fresh chemistry (add starter if necessary):	YES ☐	NO ☐
11. Clean all residue off rollers and any build-up on side plates, bearings, and gears:	YES ☐	NO ☐
12. Remove guide shoes and clean:	YES ☐	NO ☐
13. Clean drive gear, tighten screws, check springs for tension, check all o-rings (if applicable):	YES ☐	NO ☐
14. Assure processor has electrical power:	YES ☐	NO ☐
15. Verify recirculation before racks are replaced:	YES ☐	NO ☐
16. Check for proper replenishment rate:	YES ☐	NO ☐
17. Check for water flow:	YES ☐	NO ☐
18. Check for proper drainage:	YES ☐	NO ☐
19. Run several clearing films:	YES ☐	NO ☐
20. Examine films for scratches/debris and review PM/Cleaning with customer:	YES ☐	NO ☐

INDEX

Italicized numbers represent figures and tables.

ISBN 0-8385-8130-7

90000

9 780838 581308

BOONE/POCKET GUIDE
TO CHIROPRACTIC